Worry Less, Live More

Worry Less, Live More

How to Reduce Overthinking, Stress and Burnout

MICHELLE SPIRIT

ILLUSTRATIONS BY MUDD BEXLEY

Publisher: Badger Books Ltd, 2024

The moral right of Michelle Spirit to be identified as the author and compiler of this work has been asserted.

ISBN 978-1-7384522-2-4 (Print)
ISBN 978-1-7384522-3-1 (EBook)

Printed and bound by CPI Group (UK) Ltd, Croydon, CR0 4YY

Insta: @izustrations

Cover and interior illustrations by Mudd Bexley.

Book design by Principal Publishing.

Publisher website: nialledworthy.com

Email: niall@nialledworthy.com

Insta: @nialledworthybooks

To those who struggle to be kind to themselves, to find their way through the highs and lows of life and who sometimes feel like they are not enough – you are the reason this book exists. May it serve as a guide and a gentle reminder of your unique value and worth in this world.

Contents

Author's Note

There is no one-size-fits-all approach to navigating life's challenges. However, research shows what works for many. This book is designed to be your gentle companion during some of the more difficult moments. It shares simple ideas to inspire the little choices to guide you to a more hopeful, brighter path during some of the darker times. Choices that remind you to treat yourself with kindness to help reduce the overthinking, stress and anxiety that so often take hold during these times.

Michelle Spirit, Chichester, 2025

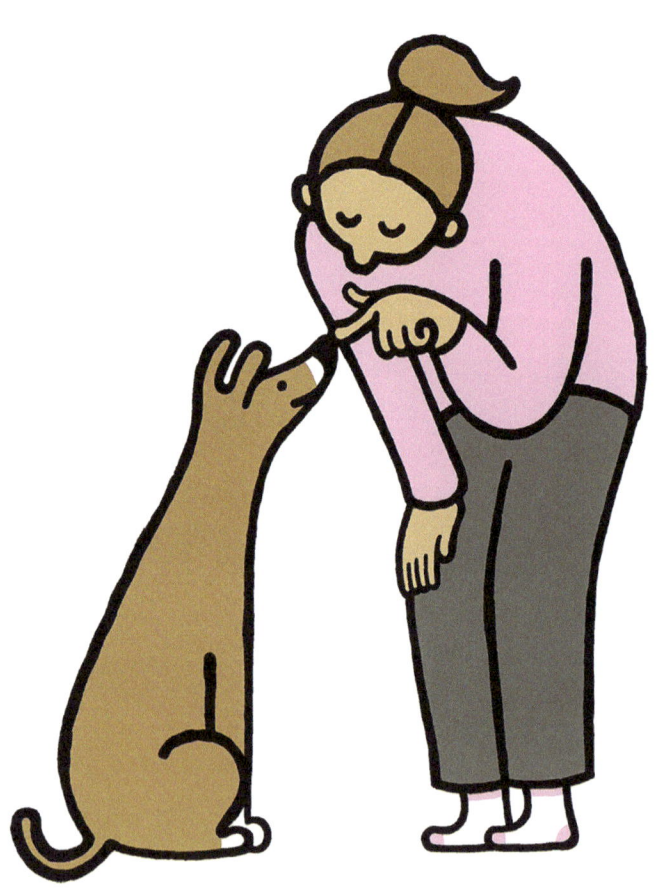

Get a (friendly!) dog

Research found a group of stockbrokers with hypertension who were given a dog to care for six months were far less stressed, with their dog ownership more effective at reducing stress than medication.[1]

Whether it's exercise, having a friendly ear or the calming effect of petting, no one really knows. What we do know is that they have a huge impact.[2] Interesting that all those stockbrokers refused to hand back their furry friend at the end of experiment. You don't have to get a real one either. Robotic dogs have been found to have had the same effect. Really.

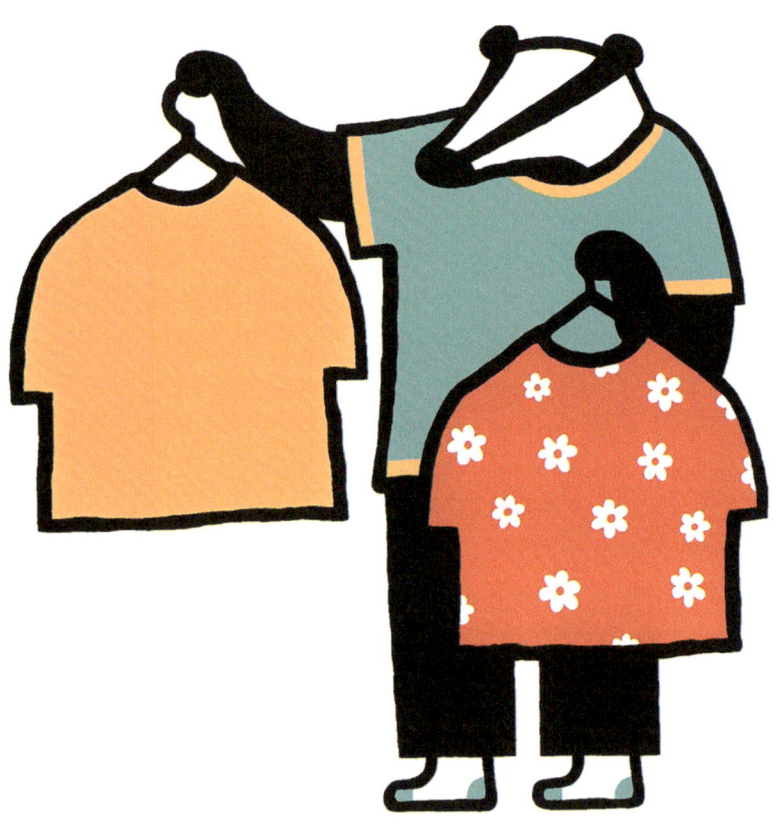

Reduce choice

Studies suggest we make 35,000 choices a day, with over 200 choices about food alone.[3] Too much choice makes us feel out of control and unhappy. Focus energy only on the decisions that really matter. When agonising over what to wear, what to watch or what to eat, stop. Ask yourself why you are putting yourself through all that stress. Stick with what you know works and save your mental energy for those really important decisions.

People are more likely to purchase luxury jams or chocolates or to undertake optional class essay assignments when offered 6 options rather than a more extensive array of 24 or 30. Moreover, participants reported greater subsequent satisfaction with their selections and wrote better essays when their original set of options had been limited.[4]

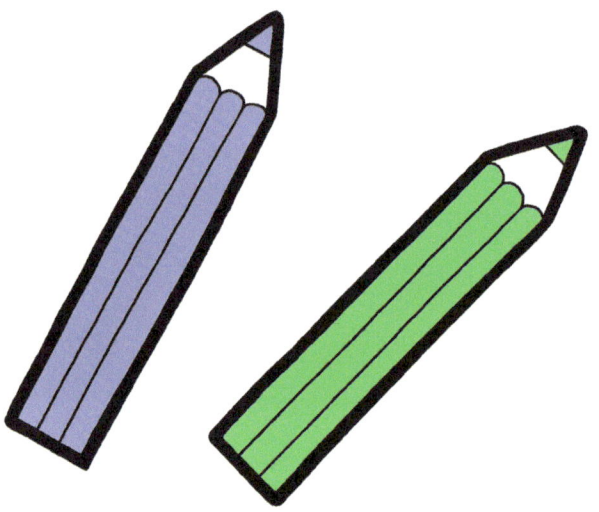

Write down your innermost thoughts and feelings

Endlessly talking or thinking about something upsetting will rarely help. Our thoughts repeat, are often disorganised and often serve only to confuse us.

Writing is more linear. Getting our thoughts and feelings down on paper offers a chance to make sense of what has happened and to figure out a way forward. Research has found that it can also make us feel happier and reduce health problems.[5]

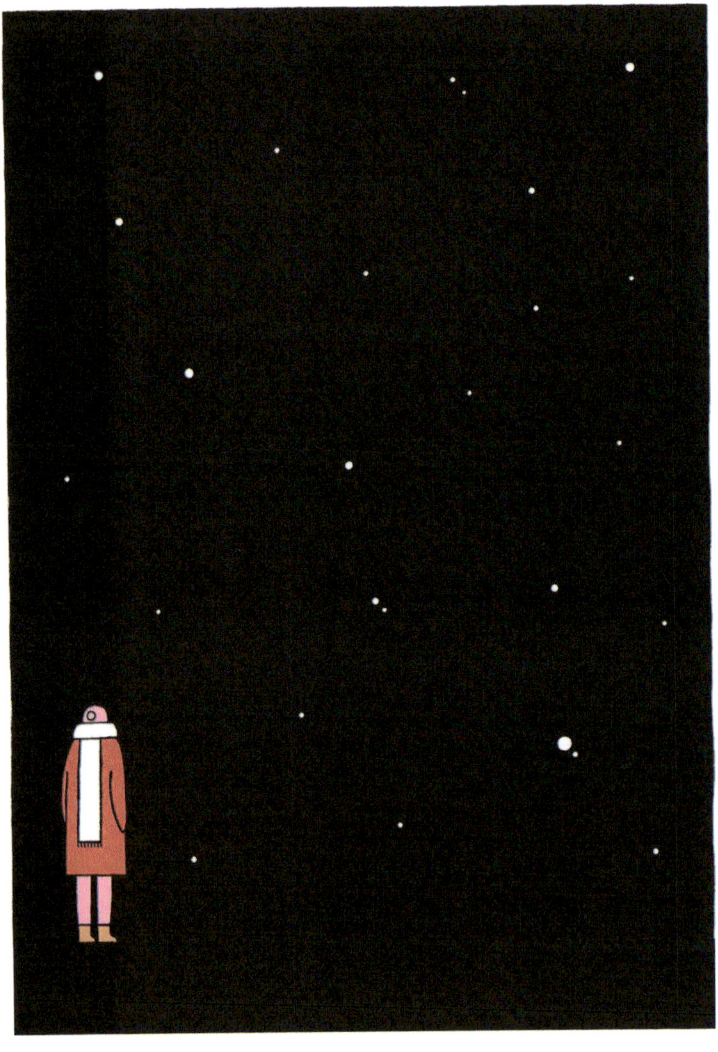

Connect to something bigger

Think how you can feel part of something bigger than your-self – through community, nature, or spiritual practices for example. This core human need really helps provide a sense of meaning and purpose to life[6], both linked to longer life expectancy and improved mental health.[7]

So how about volunteering, spending time in nature, or joining a group that shares the same values and interests as you to help deepen your relationship with yourself and the world around you?

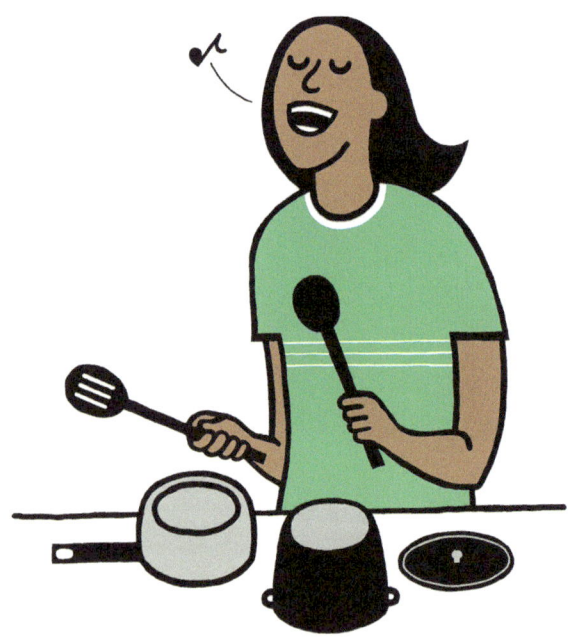

Play music, sing, dance or drum

Playing music triggers the release of endorphins which have healing qualities.[8]

So, a jive around the bedroom, belting out a rock ballad in the bath, or a good bang on the saucepans in the kitchen can have far-reaching effects. Just make sure you warn the neighbours!

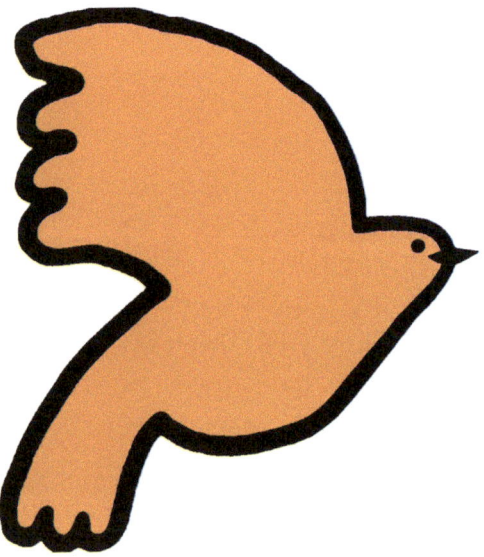

Don't play the lottery

Those who win the lottery are no more or less happy than the rest of us. The only difference is that those who don't are much better at getting pleasure from the simple things in life.

Once we have the essentials in life any increase in income seems to make little difference to our happiness.[9]

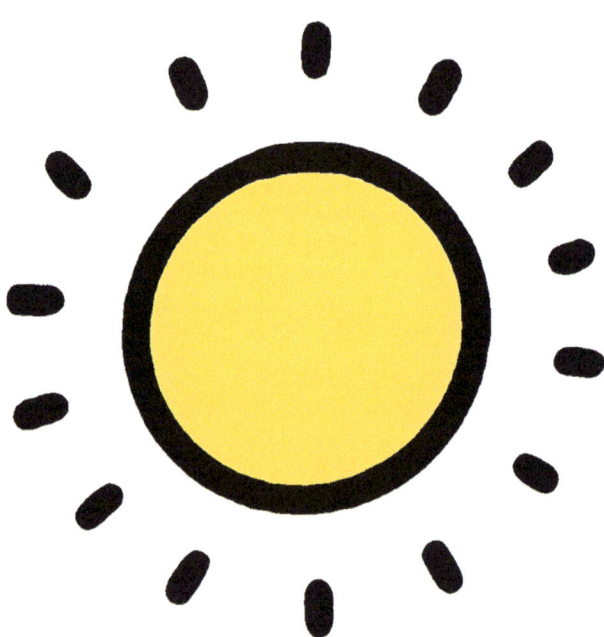

Don't try and push out negative thoughts – they'll only get worse

The more we try not to think about something the more we will think about it.

So don't tell yourself to not eat the chocolate, have the cigarette, or dwell on what upsets you about yourself. The more you tell yourself not to, the more persistently you will.

On average, people have about 60,000 to 80,000 thoughts per day, with studies indicating that approximately 70-80% of these thoughts can be negative.[10]

"I've lived through some terrible things in my life, a few of which actually happened."
Mark Twain

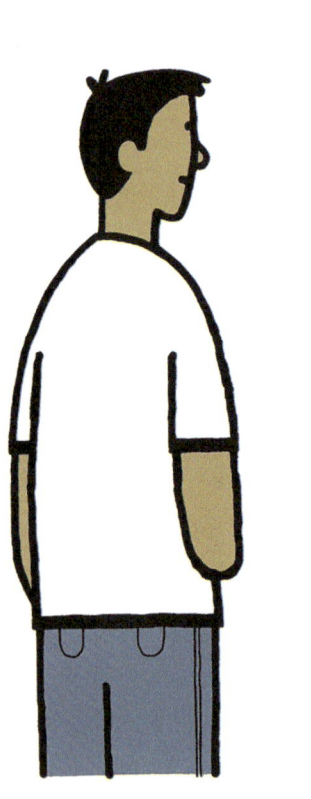
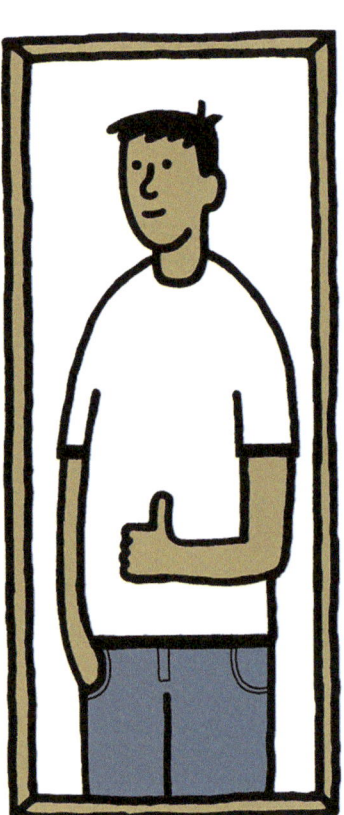

Be nice to yourself

There is a strong link between our health and how we view ourselves which affects our immune function, blood sugar and aging.[11] Sadly, many of us are often our own worst critic.[12]

Here are a couple of techniques to help grow that self-compassion muscle: Write five things you like about yourself every day in a journal. When struggling treat yourself as you would a child or friend in the same situation – paying close attention to any mean or unsupportive self-talk – really thinking, and picturing in your mind, what you would say and how.

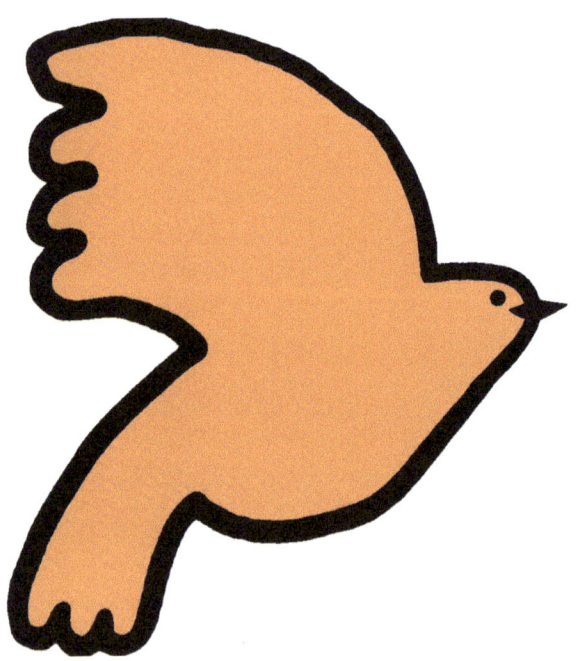

When speaking to yourself do this in the third person

This has been found to help create psychological distance, reducing feelings of inadequacy, shame and rumination.[13]

It's a mental trick that not only makes us feel better, and more in control, it also improves decision-making and performance. For instance,

"Michelle is feeling frustrated because she received a parking ticket *after* buying a ticket. Michelle wonders if the traffic warden just wanted some cardio!"

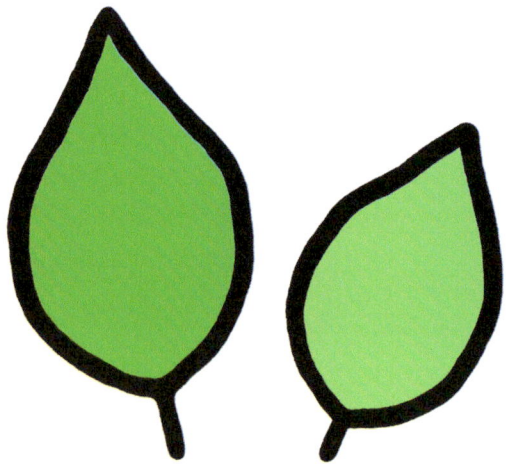

Use a compassionate voice when talking to yourself

Professor Kristen Neff, the leading authority on self-compassion, designed a programme for healthcare workers which helped them relate differently to themselves in the moment.

As a result, they experienced less stress, and anxiety and reduced rates of burnout[14]. So next time you find yourself saying 'You idiot!' when you do something you're not proud of, try a different approach that offers a fairer, kinder response such as 'this is really tough right now, I've got a lot going on'.

Nearly one in four people in the UK report high feelings of anxiety.[15]

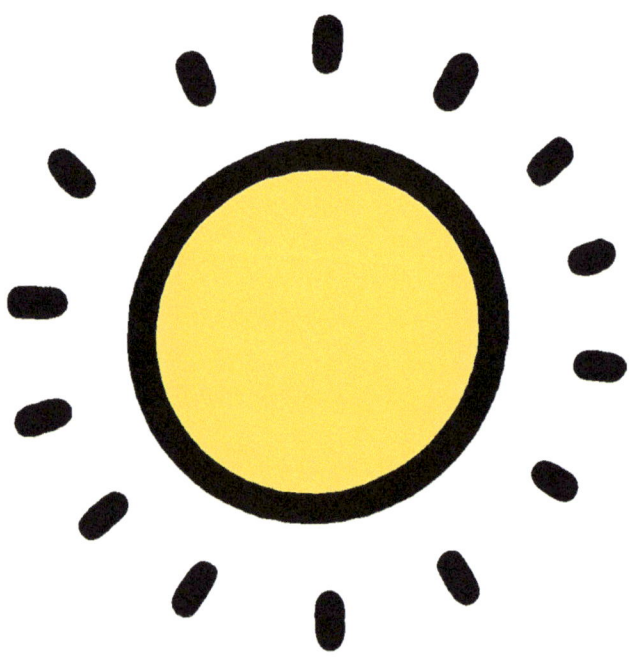

Manage criticism

No one actually *likes* to be criticised. If someone does criticise you, it has been found to be helpful to tune into how you feel, and to find a word that best describes the emotion.[16] Could be anger, frustration or fear – whatever the word, name it. Then notice where you feel the emotion in the body. Is it a tight chest, sinking feeling in your stomach, clenched jaw? Breathe deeply into this area and observe the intensity fade.

Now consider whether there is any truth in the comment. If so, is it possible to learn anything from this? If not, why might the person have said it? Consider their perspective or 'story'.

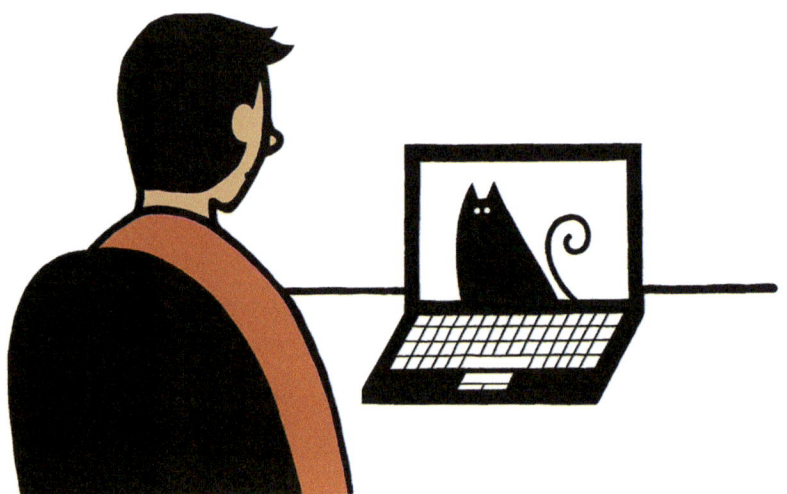

Laugh out loud
even if you don't feel like it

Laughing releases 'happy hormones', even if forced. It lifts mood, the immune system and reverses the stress response.[17]

This can help when you are struggling to see the brighter side of things, a great way of digging you out of a black mood. So, fire up those cat videos guilt-free – research shows us they really do help lift the day.

Adults typically laugh around 15 to 20 times a day, whereas children can laugh significantly more, averaging 300 to 400 times a day.[18]

Find your flow

Flow is the feeling of being completely in the moment, not fixated on the things that have happened, or that might happen. It is a mind state we enter when we are immersed in something new that interests us, that we enjoy or that we are finding slightly challenging. It's when we feel most alive, almost as if time has stood still.[19]

Studies show flow makes us 500 per cent more productive and 600 per cent more creative. Find your flow. Could be anything… Learning a challenging recipe? Brushing up your language skills? Origami? Whatever you choose, aim to do something that creates flow at least twice a week for 15 minutes.

"The best moments in our lives are not the passive, receptive, relaxing times . . . The best moments usually occur if a person's body or mind is stretched to its limits in a voluntary effort to accomplish something difficult and worthwhile."
Mihaly Csikszentmihalyi (pronounced Chick Sent Me High!)

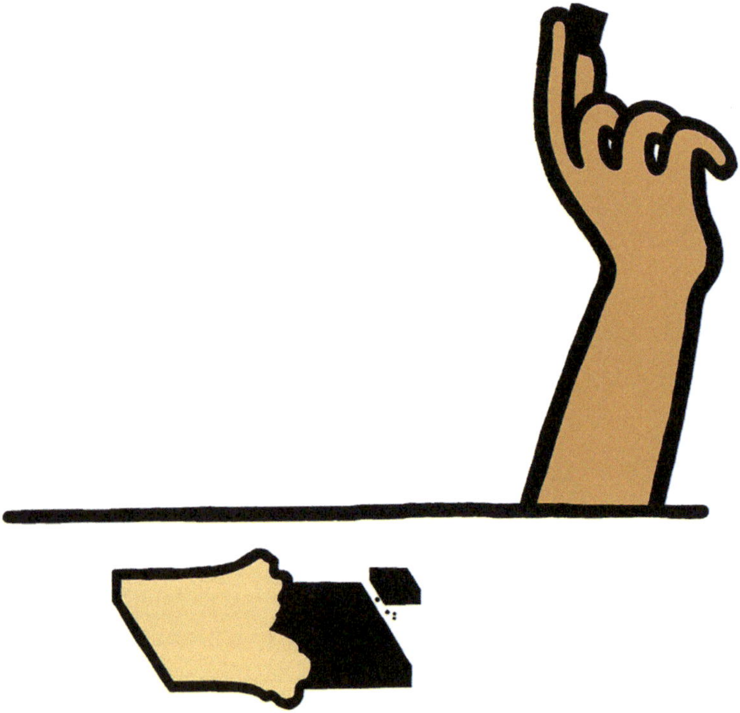

Eat some dark chocolate

This will result in part of your brain called the hypothala-
mus releasing endorphins[20] – the chemicals in the body that
reduce stress, and improve mood and sense of well-being.

This is down to the polyphenols in it – all-natural stuff
that act as antioxidants and have anti-inflammatory prop-
erties. This is why dark chocolate is better as it has more
cocoa and so more of these polyphenols. Before you tuck
into a whole bar, remember that you don't need much. Just
a few small squares can do the trick – sorry about that!

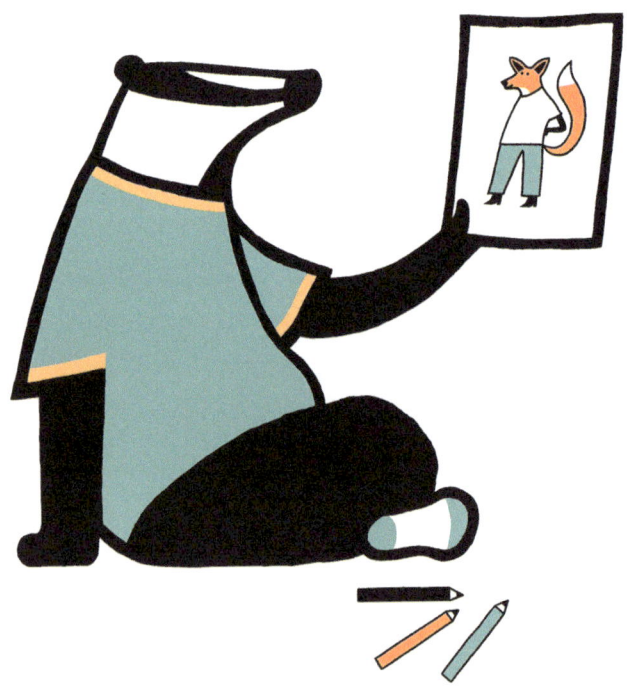

Be creative

Doing something creative reduces stress and improves feelings of well-being.[21]

As well as the more obvious writing, drawing or painting it could be as simple as drawing 20 circles on a piece of paper, and then filling them by drawing images of recognisable objects, playing with Lego or switching the way the furniture is arranged in your home.

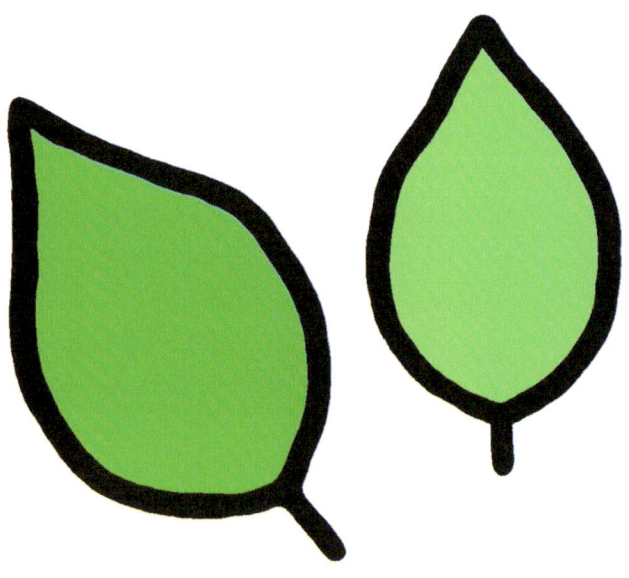

Look in the mirror

When you are getting ready for the day take the time to look at yourself in the mirror for 30 seconds. Look into your eyes and imagine you are seeing yourself through the eyes of someone who loves you (could be that dog you got!… See first tip). Smile.

Notice the qualities they appreciate in you and feel the love and warmth they have for you. Say something nice to yourself.

This will help you accept yourself for who you are and be less vulnerable to the opinions of others. It also builds confidence and feelings of self-worth.[22]

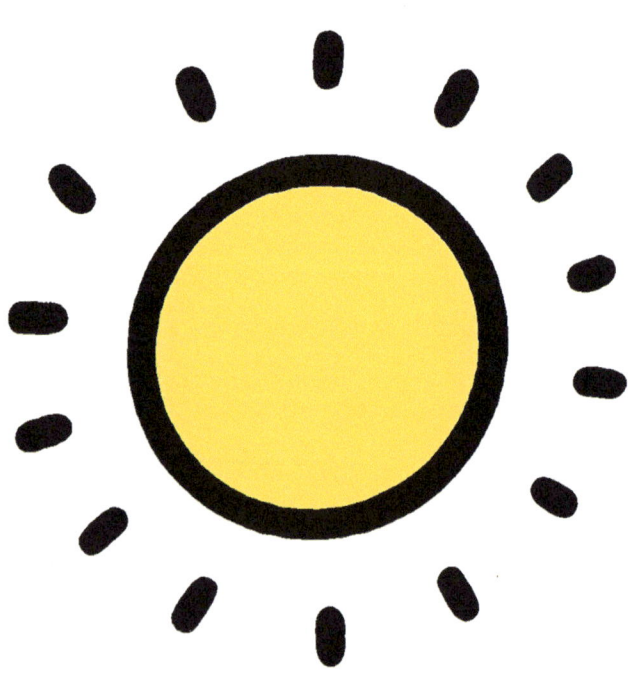

Breathe deeply

Deep diaphragmatic breathing – also known as belly breathing – has been shown to reduce stress, and lower blood pressure.[23]

Here's a simple and effective way of doing it:

1. Find a square-shaped object, such as a window, book, or even a phone screen.

2. As your eyes trace one edge of the square, inhale deeply through your nose for a count of seven, focusing on filling the belly with air like a balloon.

3. As your eyes move down the next edge, exhale slowly through your mouth for a count of eleven.

4. Repeat this pattern, moving along each edge of the square repeatedly, until you feel more relaxed and grounded.

Such a simple exercise that you can use anytime you feel overwhelmed to help you reset your focus and regain control.

The average adult takes 12 to 20 breaths per minute, which amounts to approximately 17,000 to 30,000 breaths per day.[24]

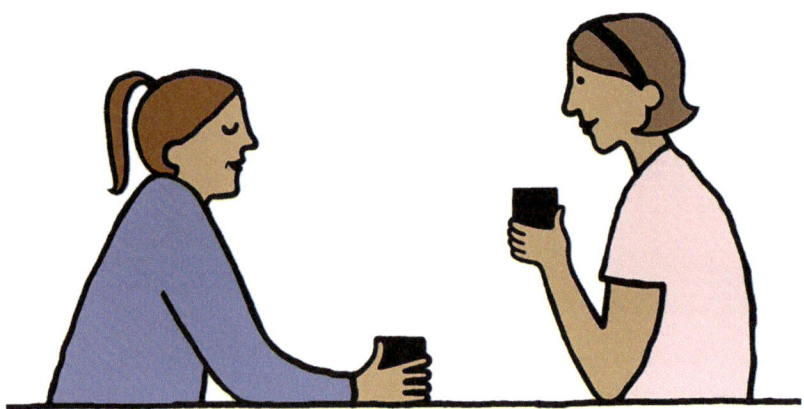

Talk things out

It's good to talk. Putting your feelings and thoughts into words with a trusted friend or family member can help you get a clearer perspective on things, feel less alone, and even boost your immune system.[25] Even the simplest conversation can make a difference. So, reach out, and find the time to grab a coffee with your trusted people.

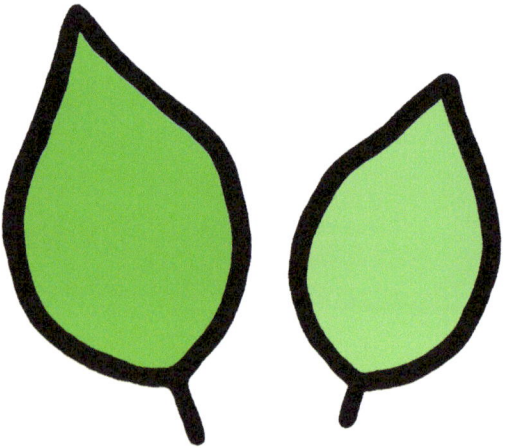

Treasure your time

Time is the most precious resource we have. Use it intentionally and guard it with your life. Use money to buy yourself time not things. Studies show that when working adults do this, they are far happier. And you don't have to be wealthy to benefit.

Professor Ashley Whillans from Harvard Business School took a group of Kenyan women who worked full-time and earned $10 a day. He split them into two groups. One received a timesaving, the other some money, both equal to three days' labour.

Both groups increased their well-being, reduced stress and noted improved relationships. However, those given timesaving reported a longer-lasting effect.[26]

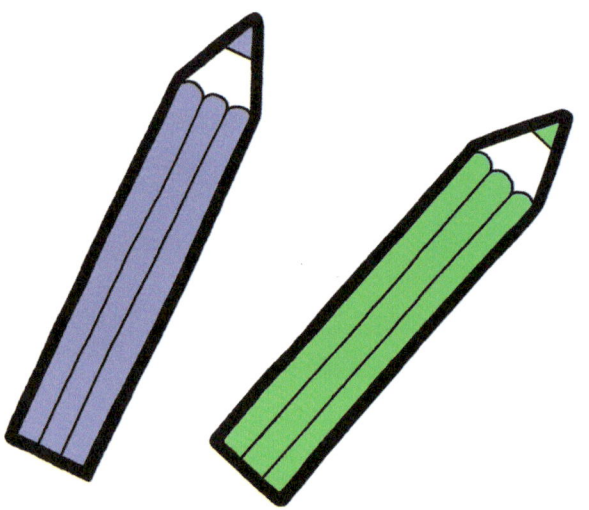

Change the story

What story are you telling yourself about your life? Changing this 'story' can deeply shape your mindset and doing so could completely transform your life. For inspiration check out John McAvoy's journey.[27]

A former career criminal, now a world record-holding athlete who saw himself as a victim of 'the system', John chose to rewrite his story whilst serving time in prison, recognising that he had this choice. Was his life of crime really a result of others? His upbringing? Changing his story changed his identity. He went on to become a world record-holding endurance athlete. Today, John inspires millions, showing that it's never too late to create a more empowering narrative.

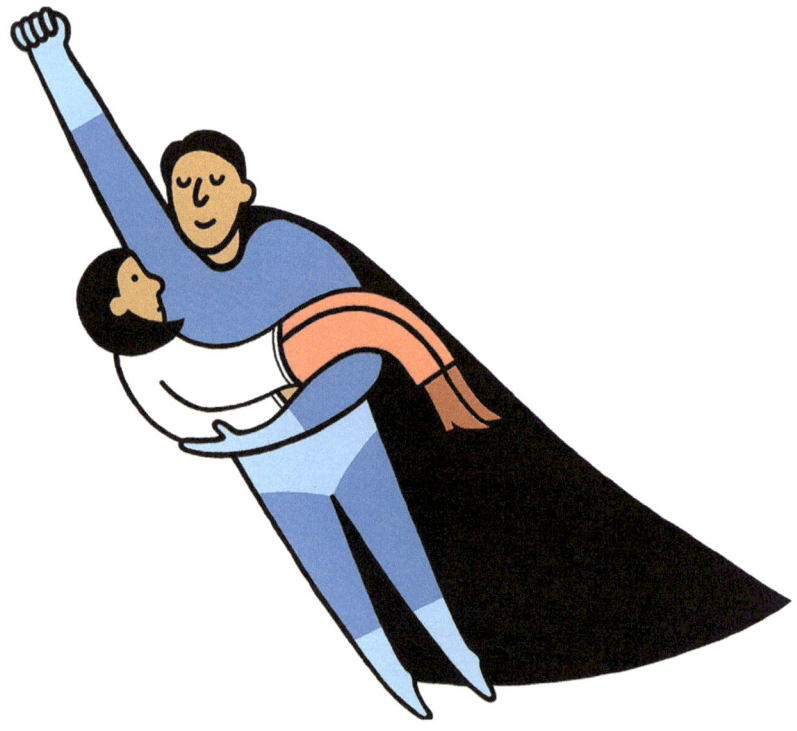

Stop being the victim

Do you have a strong reaction to small hurts or injustices done to you? Believe you are much more conscientious and moral in your relations with others compared to their treatment of you? Yes? You might then have a tendency to interpersonal victimhood.[28] This could be making you feel powerless, out of control and frankly exhausted.

To heal, try telling others your thoughts and feelings in the moment rather than pushing them down. Start asking directly for what you want and need. Reflect on whether you are helping others because they truly need support or because it makes you feel better about yourself.

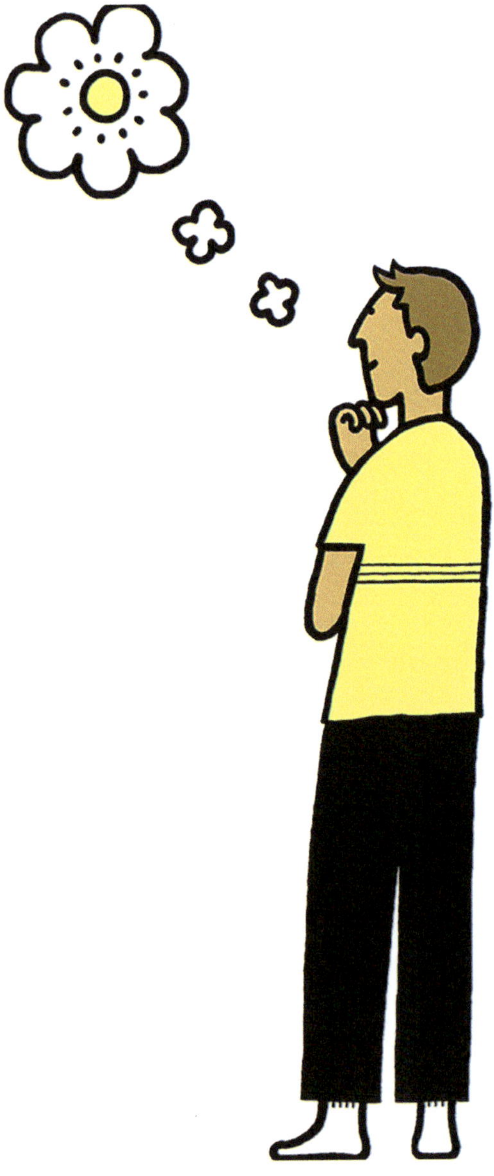

Choose your thoughts

Dr Edith Egar, a holocaust survivor and renowned psychologist, shares her extraordinary journey of survival, healing, and forgiveness, advising us to 'embrace our power to choose', and that even in the most desperate of times we can choose our thoughts, attitudes and responses.[29]

Which means that even in the darkest of moments we can decide what we focus on and our response. Her wisdom encourages us to recognise that freedom.

So try to stop trusting that what you think is always the truth – remember that we often tune into the more negative of perceptions, we just can't help ourselves. But know that we do this and that only by gently tuning into our thoughts, and observing and questioning them, can we really change our response to life's challenges.

"What a liberation to realise that the 'voice in my head' is not who I am. Who am I then? The one who sees that."
Eckhart Tolle

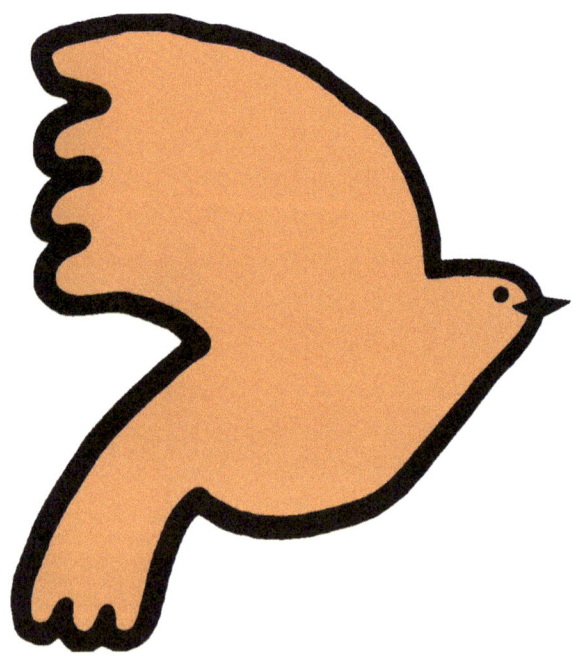

Spend on experiences, not stuff

Research has found that the excitement of buying fades, but the joy and memories of experiences last way longer, sometimes even a lifetime.[30]

A new Porsche might be fun for a while, but doing things that bring you joy, especially if you do them with or for others, will have a much bigger impact in the longer term.[31] So, take a trip, try a new hobby or learn something new. Experiences trump possessions.

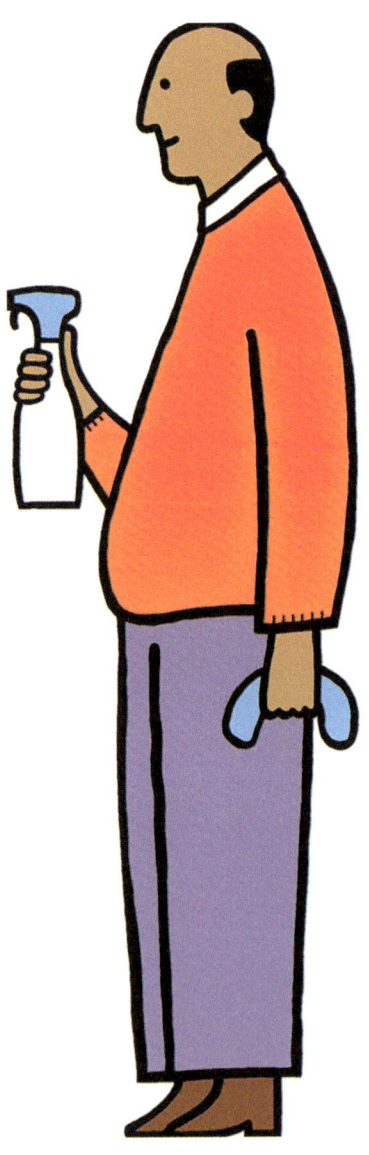

Give

Few ways provide a more powerful boost than giving.[32]

So, when you are trying to cheer yourself up by scrolling through websites or wandering around shops for that new outfit/jewellery/gadget for yourself, switch your attention to what you might buy for someone else… a surprise gift for a loved one maybe?

Perhaps instead of a material 'thing' you could give them the gift of time by paying for someone to valet their car, clean the house or look after the kids so they get a night out with their loved one.

Get this – the joy of giving and receiving isn't equated to how much the gift costs. As little as £5 has been found to make both the giver and receiver happier regardless of how much financial wealth they have.

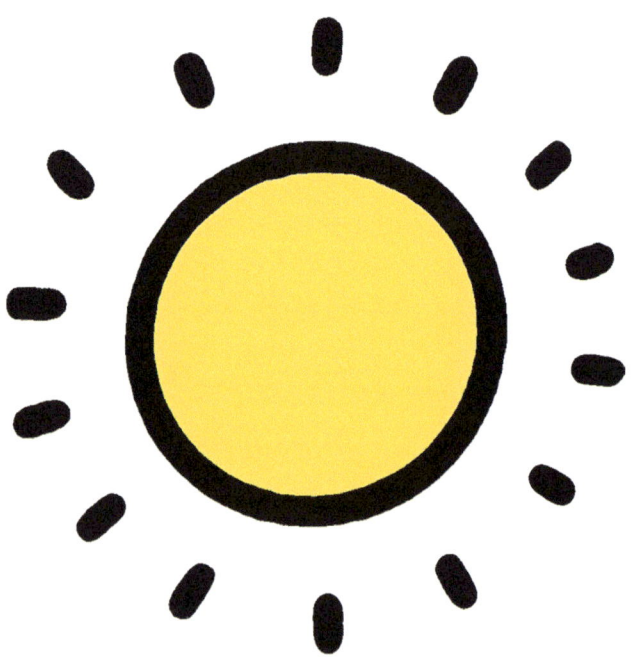

Have one quality conversation with a friend daily

This will make you happier and less stressed.[33] The conversation could be a catch-up, a joke shared or simply to let them know that you are thinking of them. Face to face is of course better than electronic or social media, but anything is better than nothing when it comes to catching up with our friends.

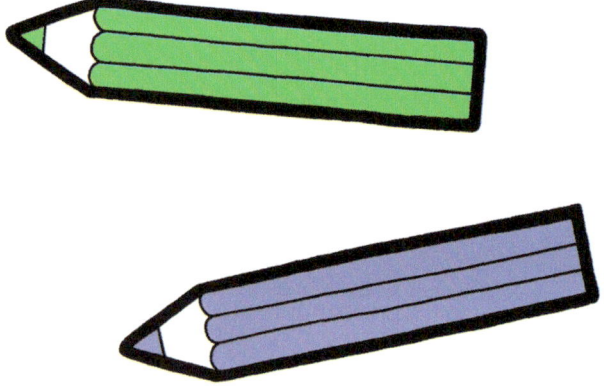

Label your feelings

Whenever you have strong negative feelings label them. Otherwise, you risk getting swept along in a wave of confusion and sorrow, or even pushing those feelings deeper down into your heart, where at some point they will no doubt erupt uncontrollably.

What feelings are you experiencing? Sadness? Frustration? Anger? Labelling them activates the parts of the brain that deal with language and meaning, which moves us away from feelings of suffering as it reduces the brain's fight or flight reaction.[34]

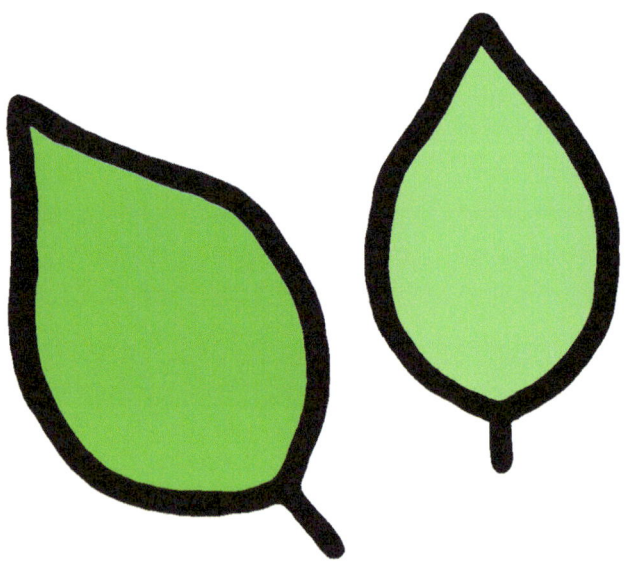

Stop procrastinating, start the task

If you are a chronic procrastinator – and 24% of us are – you increase the risk of anxiety[35], so for a few minutes, just tell yourself to start the task. So often we are put off by the sheer size of the project we don't even attempt to get going on it.

However, we also dislike tasks being only partially completed so chances are once you've started something you will feel compelled to keep going!

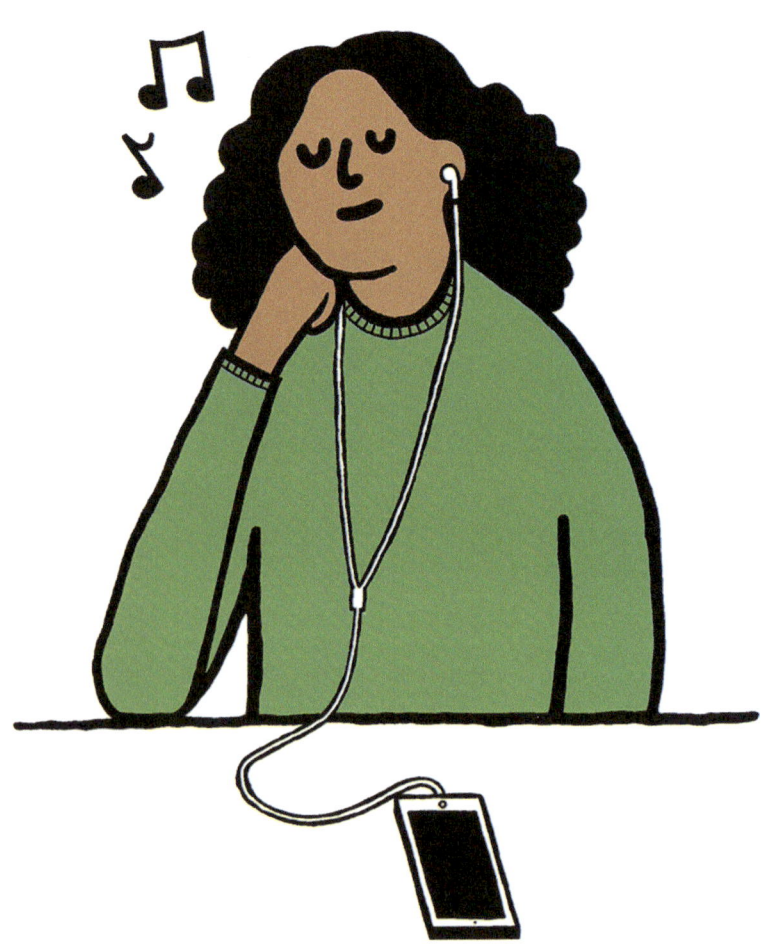

Listen to classical music

This affects the autonomic nervous system and vagus nerve which responds to musical vibrations, leading to a relaxation response.[36] Fast music can also affect our mood through the release of neurotransmitters such as dopamine. Music then has the power to speed up our heart rate and slow it down. So, dial it up, or dial it down as the situation requires!

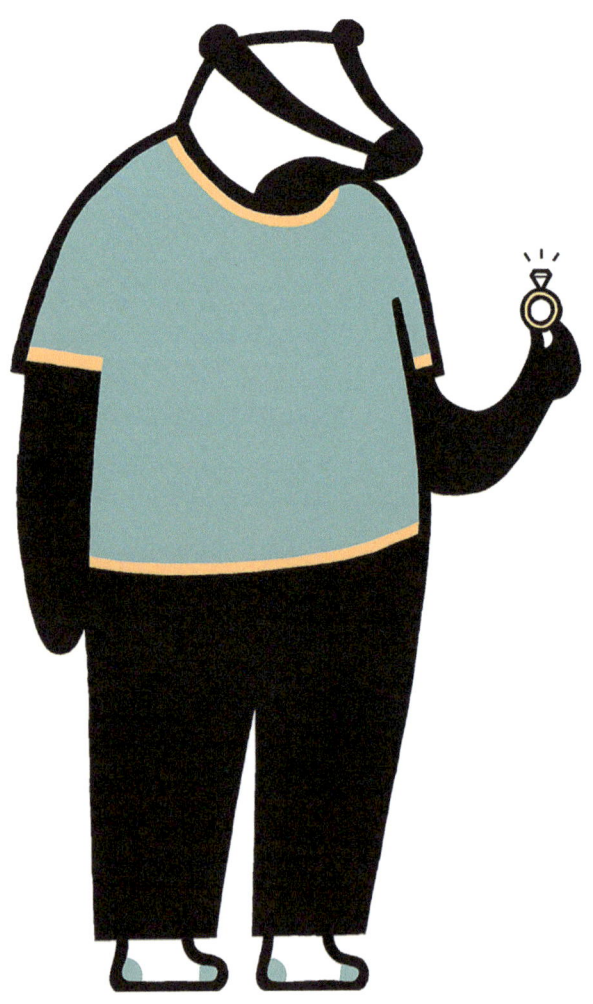

Lose the idea that marriage is the answer

Whilst the average couple, in the months before marriage, experience generally improving mental and physical health, this is followed by a flattening or drop in the gains afterwards.

Studies have found there to be no sustained improvements in mental and physical well-being other than those first few months leading up to marriage.[37]

The happy fairytale ending of the prince and princess getting wed it seems is not one we should necessarily aspire to. It seems it is just that. A fairytale.

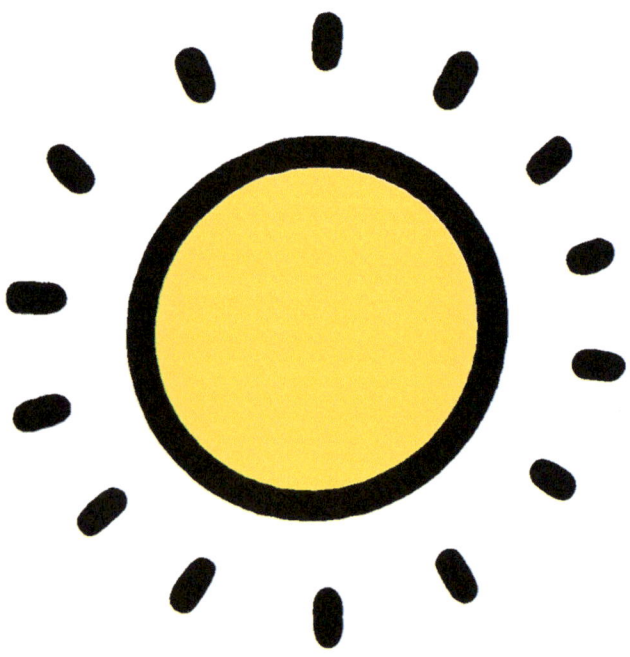

Focus on what you can control

Write a list of *all* the things that concern you. Now, strike a line through those you can do nothing about. Take a look at the remaining ones as this is where you need to focus your energy.

Practice noticing when you are dwelling on those things you put a line through, the things you have no control over. This happens to us all. A lot. Our minds are designed to wander to the bad stuff, and they do it when we are not thinking about anything in particular.[38]

When you do, stop. Breathe. Try and gently bring those thoughts back to where you want them to be. Try to get some support to help you let go and have faith in what will be when it comes to those things you can do nothing about.

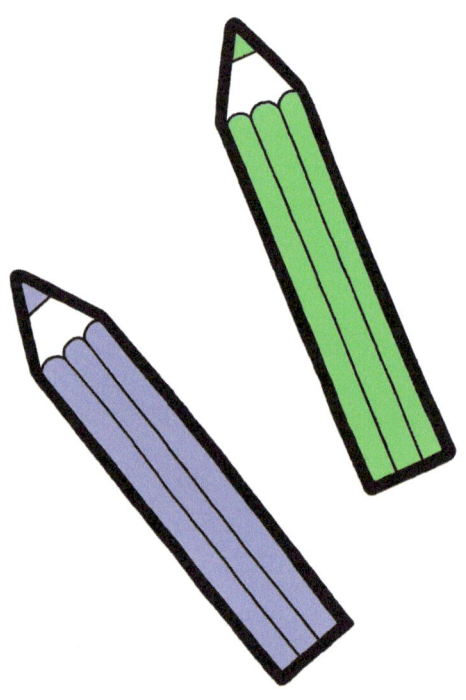

Plan for action

Gabriele Oettingen's two decades of research resulting in her WOOP model provide us with a great way of helping us feel more effective and able to reach our goals. However small these goals are this is a great way of feeling better about ourselves.[39] Here it is:

Take something on the list of things you can control or influence in some way as above, and then follow this process:

Identify your **W**ish. Then really think about what's going to feel great about achieving this – the **O**utcome. What will others notice is different about you? Next consider the **O**bstacles. What that can be controlled might get in the way of achieving that wish? Make sure you think about things that are going to be down to you and those external to you. Then finally, if they do get in the way what are you going to do about them. What is your **P**lan to overcome them?

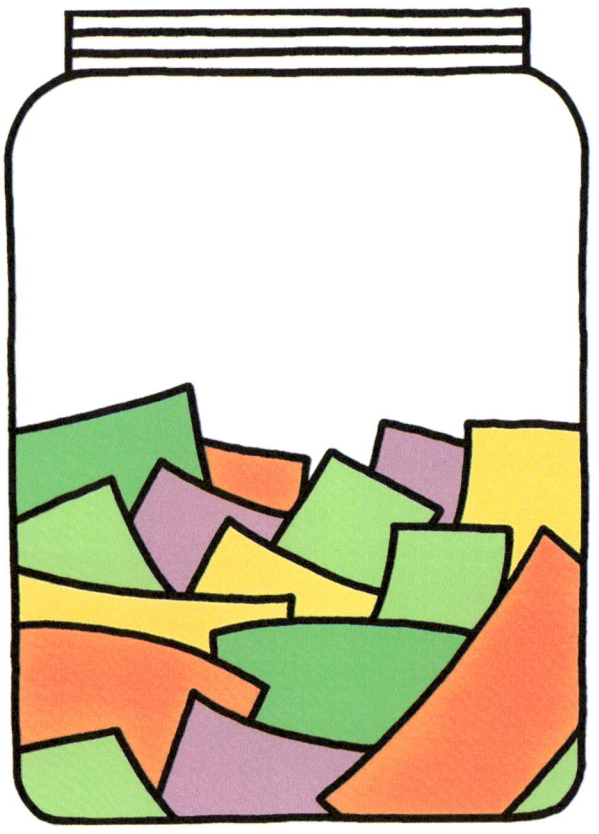

Practice gratitude

Doing this has been proven by numerous studies to have a huge impact on our mental health.[40] [41] It's simple and there are loads of ways of doing it.

Here are some ideas to play with:

- Write down five things you are grateful for each day in a journal.
- Go for a walk and take note of the sights, sounds, tastes, smells and sensations around you.
- Close your eyes and bring to your mind's eye things, you are grateful for.
- Write down the things you are grateful for on slips of paper and put them in a jar.
- Write to someone who has had a big impact on your life.
- Slow down and take in the little moments in life, the feel of the sun on your skin, the taste of something or the sound of music.

All of these train the muscle of attention to focus on what's okay rather than what's not. A powerful practice.

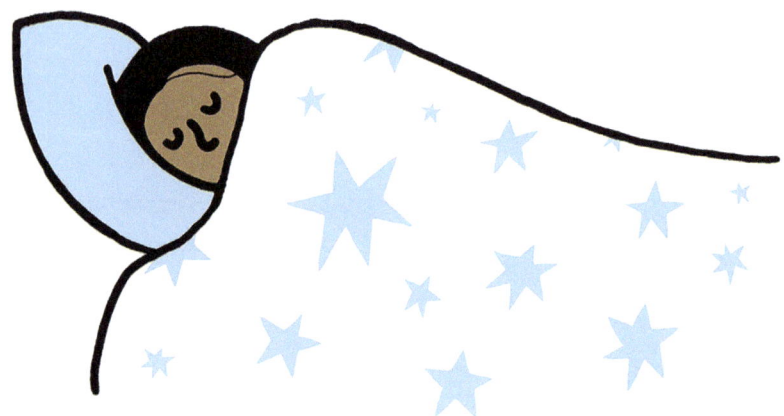

Sleep well

Ah, the foundation for health and wellness! But with a third of adults worldwide suffering from some symptoms of insomnia, sleep is a challenge for many.[42] Here are some science-based tips proven to help those who struggle to get those ZZZs.

Create a routine that includes chilling out an hour before you go to bed. Dim light, avoid screens and do something relaxing like having a bath or listening to music. Use a low red night light if you do have to get up in the night as this has the least impact on your circadian clock, and make sure you see daylight for 20 minutes first thing in the morning.

Don't have any caffeine after midday – 25 per cent of this will still be in your system 12 hours later, and it's also a good idea to avoid anything likely to trigger stress hormones before you go to bed, so save those tricky conversations for the morning.

Insomnia is associated with poorer self-rated life satisfaction, and it is estimated that individuals with insomnia would be willing to trade approximately 14 per cent of their annual per capita household income to avoid its negative consequences. That's more than they would be prepared to pay to not suffer from asthma or diabetes.[43]

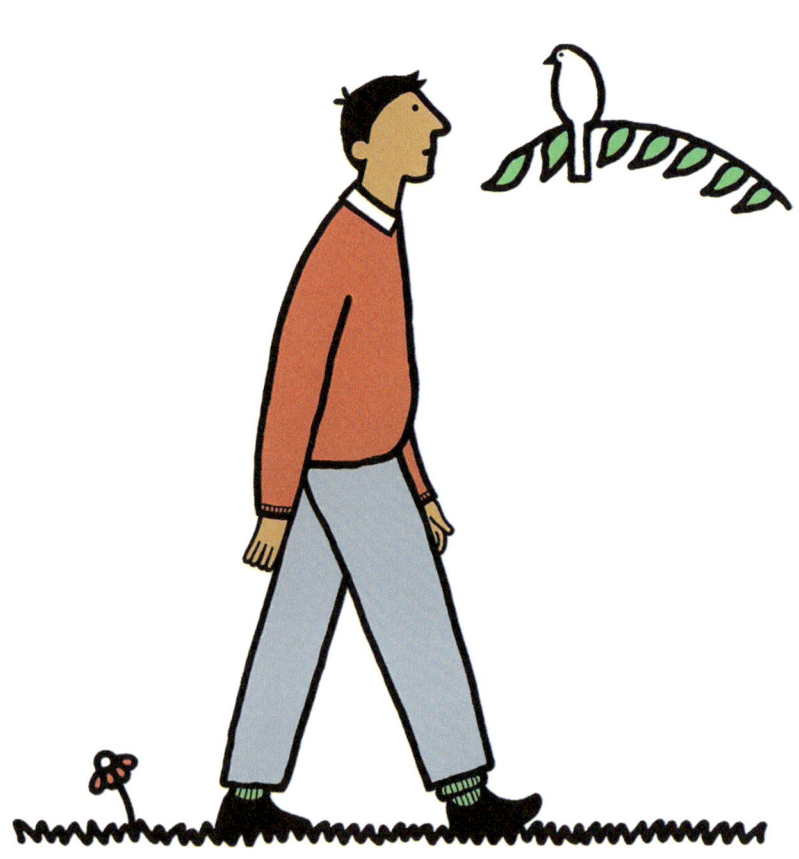

Don't get used to the good stuff

Step outside of your experience to appreciate it to improve your mood.[44] Savour the positive moments.

This could be as simple as sharpening your senses when out for a walk, thinking, 'Love that sky today!', soaking in a warm bath, spending time with a good friend or taking a mental photograph of something you want to remember. This one has the added benefit that you can revisit that memory when you are feeling a bit down.

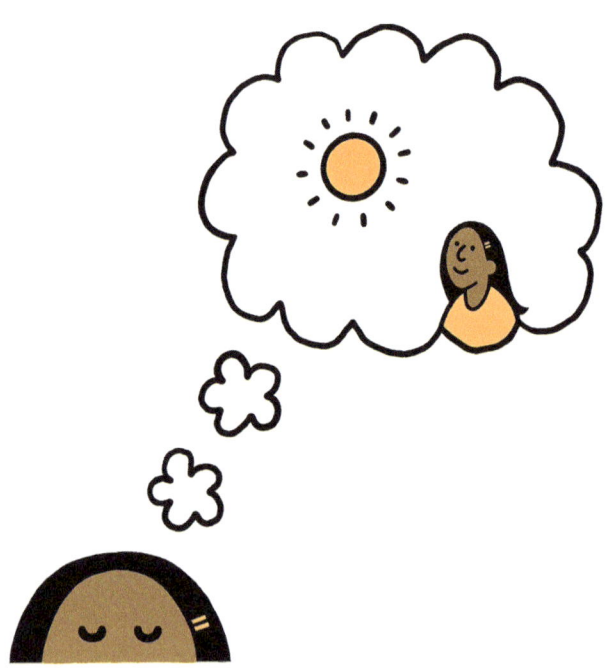

Take a trip down memory lane

Replay happy memories in your mind as if you are rewinding a video and playing it back. Try and use all your senses as if you were there.

Doing this for eight minutes a day for just three days was found to result in sustained increases in positive emotions three weeks later.[45] People who savour and reminisce about happy events in their lives feel a lot less stressed than those who don't. It's also a great way of interrupting negative thoughts.

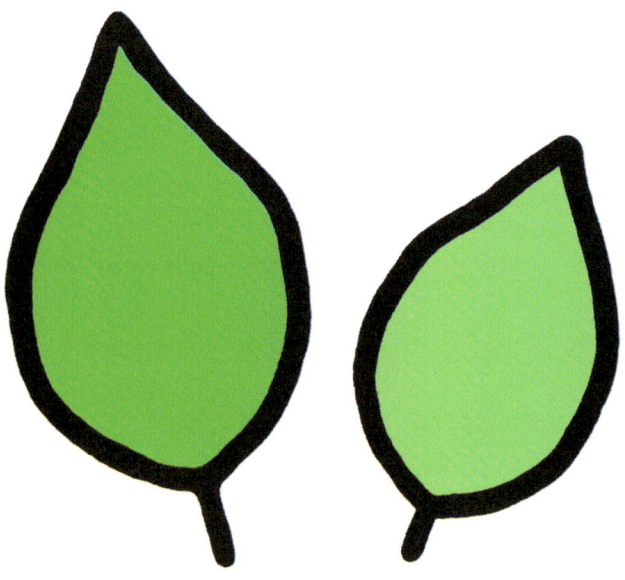

Try meditating

This can literally change your brain.[46]

It increases activity in the left prefrontal cortex, the part associated with positive thoughts, feelings, and emotions. It also decreases activity in the amygdala, which is associated with negative thoughts and emotions.

Even more importantly, it stops the brain's annoying tendency to drift off and focus on the bad stuff.[47] There are loads of different ways of meditating – mindfulness meditation, progressive muscle relaxation, guided visualisation and loving-kindness meditation[48] to name but a few.

While the average adult breathes about 12 to 20 times per minute, experienced meditators may reduce their breathing rate to about 6 to 10 breaths per minute during meditation practices.[49]

Find some benefit in the face of adversity

When thinking about something bad that has happened, instead of running the negatives over in your mind, turn your attention to the benefits of the event. Try and dig into why you found the situation so difficult.

What does it teach you about yourself? Focus on other benefits. Did you become wiser? Stronger? This technique is proven to help with frustration, anger and/or sorrow following a negative event. It also makes us more forgiving and less likely to seek retribution.[50]

By middle age, the average person is likely to have 3-5 significant life challenges (such as job loss, illness, or family issues).[51]

"If someone comes along and shoots an arrow into your heart, it's fruitless to stand there and yell at the person. It would be much better to turn your attention to the fact that there's an arrow in your heart."
Pema Chödrön

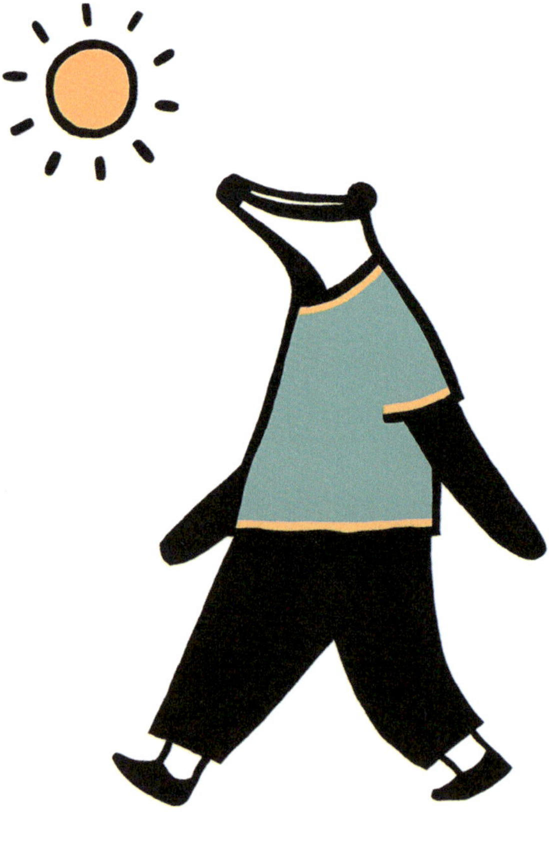

Limit screen time

In the UK, we spend on average 7 hours and 20 minutes looking at a screen a day, 3 hours and 28 minutes on our smartphones alone.[52]

Too much of this, especially social media showing us filtered images and wondrous lives, most of which are fake, makes us feel we are not enough, anxious and fed up.[53] Stop comparing yourself to others, as this will only drain energy and make you feel you are lacking in some way.[54]

Set boundaries by having a place where devices live, and have designated screen-free times in the day – during a meal maybe, or at bedtime. Start small. Do things that don't involve screens like reading, spending time outdoors, and chatting with others. Unfollow accounts that don't make you feel happy.

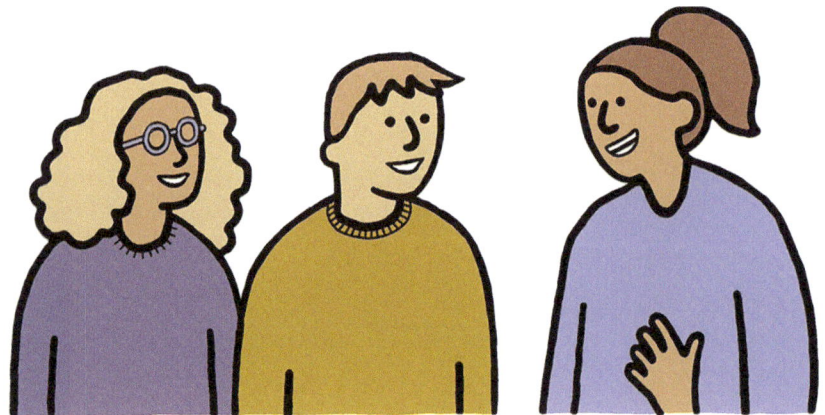

Invest time in social connections

Instead of looking at the pretend lives of others, invest time in social connections instead.

We are social beings, and we all need company to feel a sense of belonging, and to have people we can turn to for emotional support. Put time aside to call, meet up or even send a quick message as all these actions can strengthen friendships.

Volunteer at a school, charity or hospital or arrange to see your friends for a day out. To build good connections two things will help: the 1:2 rule... 1) speak about the person you meet with twice as much as you do about yourself, and 2) remember the 'if you want a friend, be a friend' principle. Don't try and impress potential friends, focus on helping them feel good about themselves instead.

Research shows a strong link between our social connections and our longevity and mental health, particularly during stressful times.[55] To motivate you, remember that the person you are befriending could be as much in need of friendship as you are!

1 in 4 adults globally report feeling very or fairly lonely. [56]

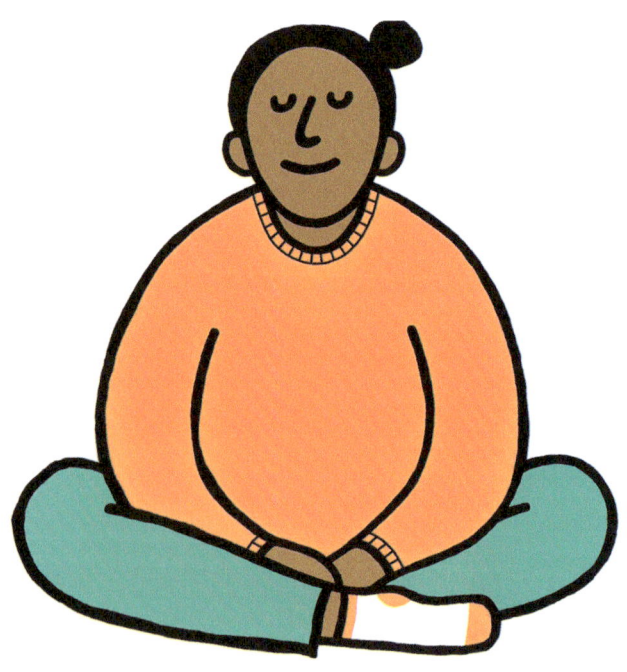

Do nothing for 15 minutes

Stress is not bad. Getting stuck feeling stressed is. It leads to chronic stress and burnout.

The good news is that just fifteen minutes of rest helps us exit the stress cycle. This is as important as what we eat, and how much we exercise and sleep, to our wellbeing. So put those all-important minutes in your diary and prioritise them. It could be as simple as a walk in the park, colouring in or reading a magazine.

What it is matters less than making sure that this is something that's just for you, doesn't involve a screen and that you feel zero guilt.

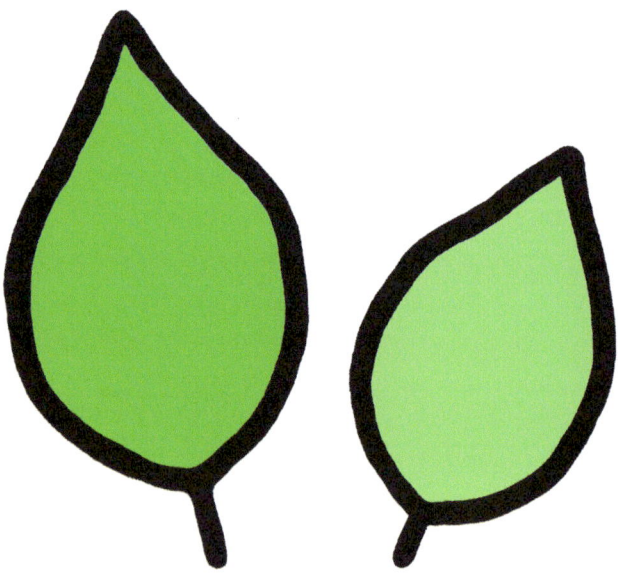

Complete the stress cycle

Our brains struggle to know the difference between real danger, and psychological danger, like rejection. It responds in the same way to both.

However, this energy-sapping response is designed solely for situations that have a quick outcome – death or life. The challenge is that psychological stressors – not getting on with your boss, money worries, kids in trouble at school, for example, don't have that black and white ending. They can indeed feel never-ending. This means we get stuck in the stress cycle. This hugely increases the risk of burning out or developing a mental health issue.[57] We can escape by belly breathing, moving, doing something creative, laughing, giving or receiving affection, crying or connecting with others.

76% of employees reported experiencing burnout at some point in their careers, with 28% stating they felt burned out "very often" or "always." [58]

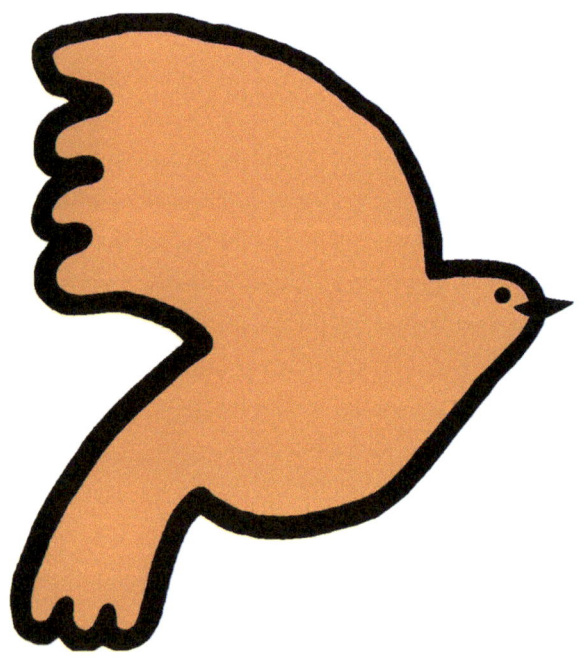

Approach news items with caution

We aren't always good at remembering that what we see on the news isn't what the majority of the people in the world are experiencing[59]. A lot focuses on aggression, selfishness and greed as those stories grab our attention. Seeing so much of this can lead us to thinking that this is how the world really is, even though it's not true.

When we keep watching these stories, it can make us act in similar ways and believe that being unkind or selfish is normal. It can also make us feel less trusting of others and less connected to the people around us. This is a problem because we need trust and kindness especially to help us through hard times.

'We are not rational enough to be exposed to the press'
Nassim Taleb

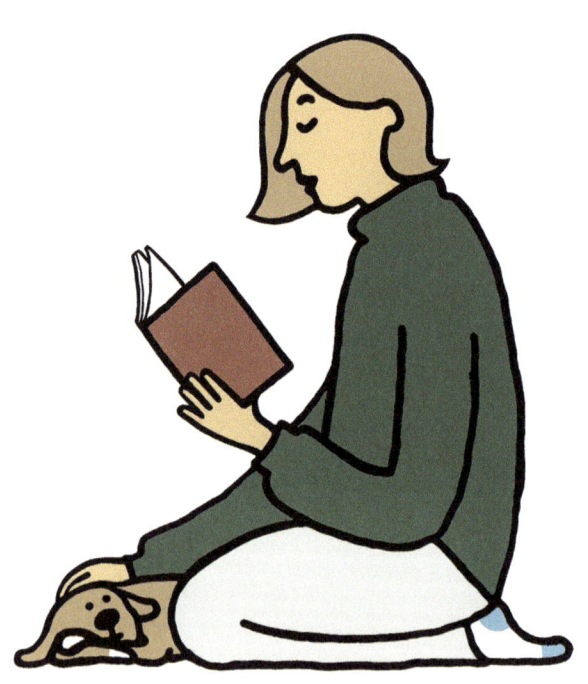

Keep learning – you CAN teach an old dog new tricks

We can rewire our brains at any age, and it's really good to shuffle those synapses around a bit.[60]

Research shows it improves cognitive functioning, minimises memory loss, boosts confidence, makes us feel less lonely, happier and gives us a sense of purpose.[61]

So, try something new or rediscover a past interest. Learn to make stuff, read a new journal, listen to a podcast. It doesn't have to be anything major, just finding a new function on your phone/cooker/TV counts. Maybe you could do something different at work or home, learn a language or make a new, challenging meal. Just make sure it's something you are interested in.

The brain processes information faster than a computer: Although it weighs only about 3 pounds, the human brain can process information at speeds estimated at up to 120 meters per second. This enables complex thought processes, emotional responses, and decision-making in mere milliseconds, which goes to show just how powerful and efficient the brain is.[62]

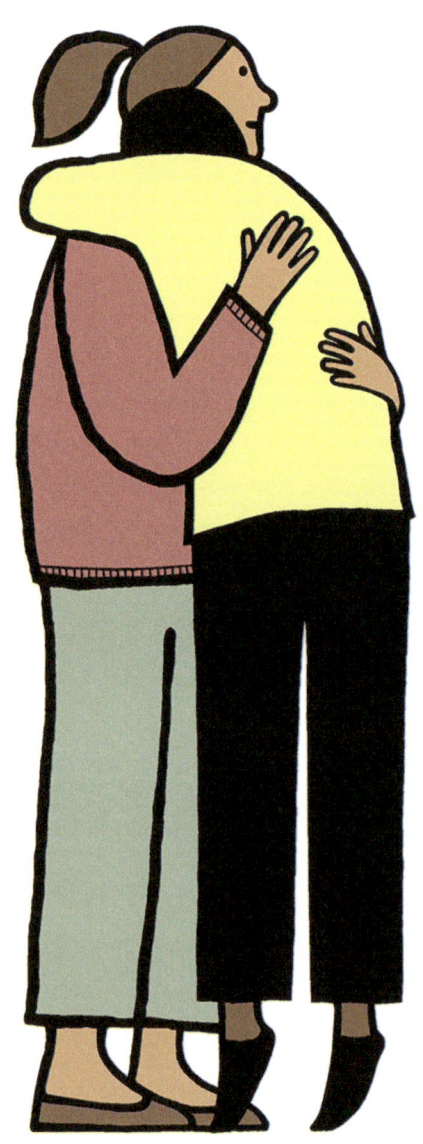

Forgive yourself and others

This can release negative emotions about yourself and others which reduces stress, anger, anxiety and depression.[63] [64] Make a note of something it would be good to forgive yourself or others for.

Perhaps a past mistake, or a behaviour of another person towards you. Acknowledge the hurt, take the perspective of the other person or yourself at the time, commit to letting go of resentment and try and see what you learnt from the situation. Writing a letter of forgiveness to a person who hurt you (even if you don't send it) can also really help.

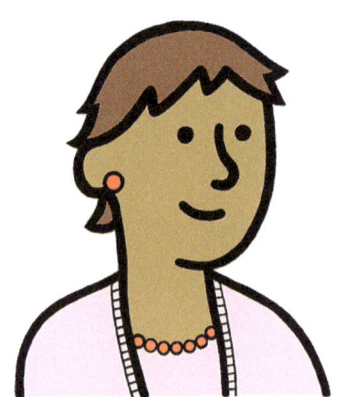
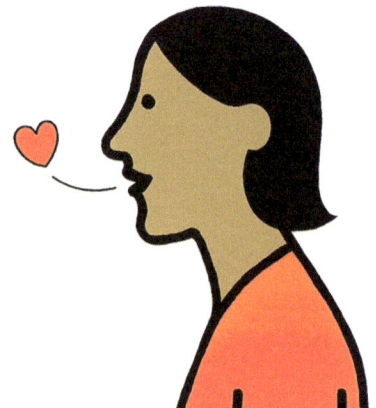

Find strength in vulnerability

Showing our vulnerability helps us emotionally connect with ourselves and others, builds trust, and empathy and makes relationships far more meaningful. It also builds self-compassion and reduces feelings of shame.[65]

If you struggle with this start by sharing small meaningful parts of yourself with trusted people, take a small emotional risk – like expressing your feelings, sharing personal stories, admitting you are wrong, asking for help or giving someone a compliment.

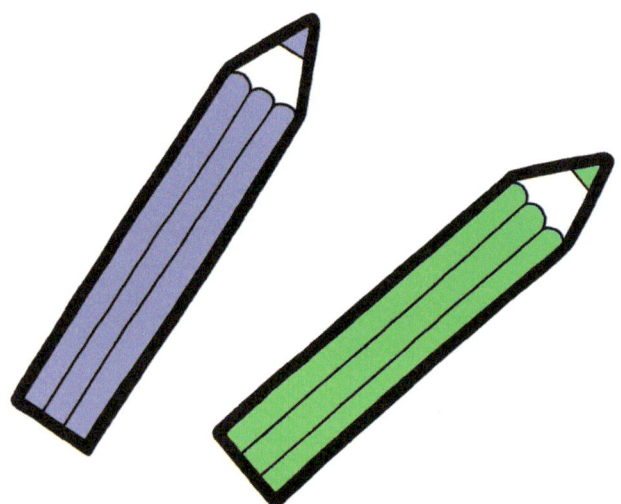

Set boundaries

Having boundaries can help all of us hang onto our emotional energy, stop us burning out, keep friendships intact and achieve a good work-life balance.[66] They make it easier to prioritise our needs which means more balanced emotions.

Start by finding a low-pressure situation where you can practice phrases like, "I appreciate the offer but I'm going to pass" or, "I can't commit to that right now". Use statements like, "I need some time to recharge so won't be able to make it this time." Keep it calm, be assertive and don't over-explain!

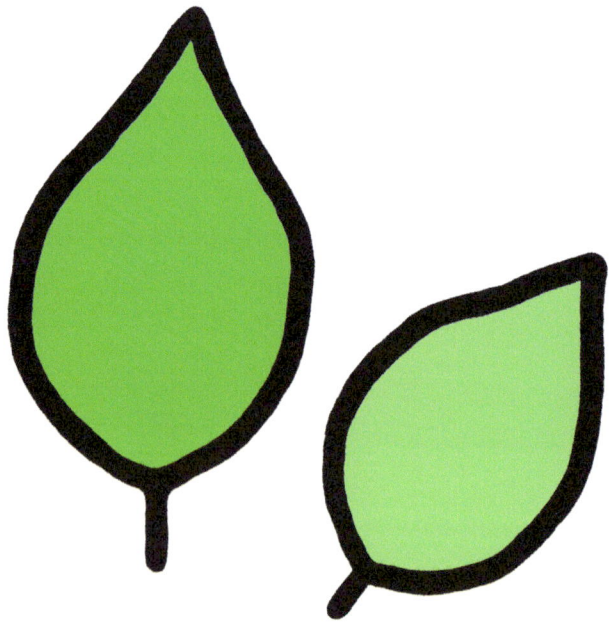

Fail

Winning feels great. Failing often feels bad. However, those who see failure as having some kind of value – a learning opportunity for example – have far lower levels of stress and anxiety.[67]

To fail well, adopt a growth mindset by seeing FAIL as your "First Attempt In Learning". Failing really is one of the best ways of learning. So reflect on the lessons you learnt and how you can improve next time rather than how bad you feel not getting it right first time.

Remember that for most of us, quiet failure is far more common than never-ending success – we just don't get to hear so much about those experiences!

Failure is common for many successful entrepreneurs with them experiencing an average of 3.8 failures before achieving lasting success.[68]

"That which does not kill us makes us stronger".
Friedrich Nietzsche.

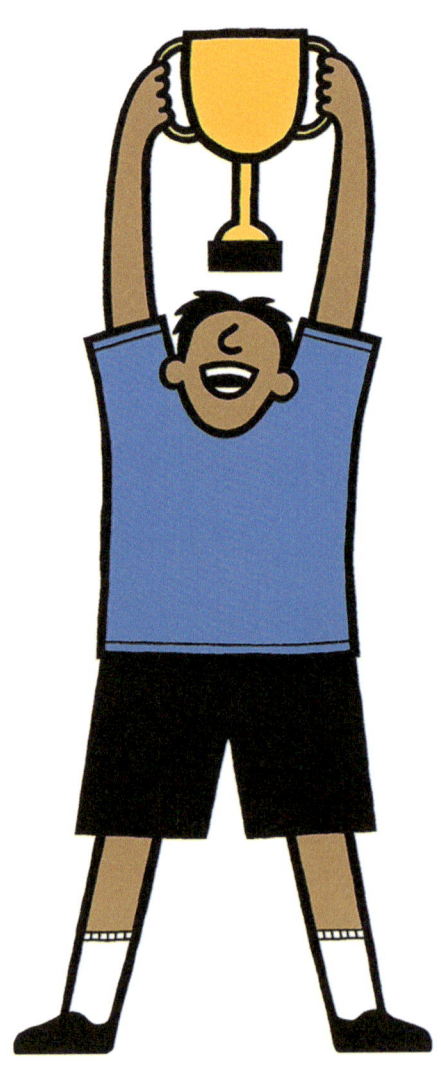

Do what you are good at

This will make you happier, and research shows that when you focus on what you're good at, you feel more positive and less stressed.[69]

Don't spend all your time trying to fix your weaknesses — building on your strengths will help you grow faster and enjoy what you're doing more. So, find what you're naturally good at, or just love doing, and find a way to use that strength every day.

"He who has a 'why' to live for, can bear almost any 'how'."
Friedrich Nietzsche

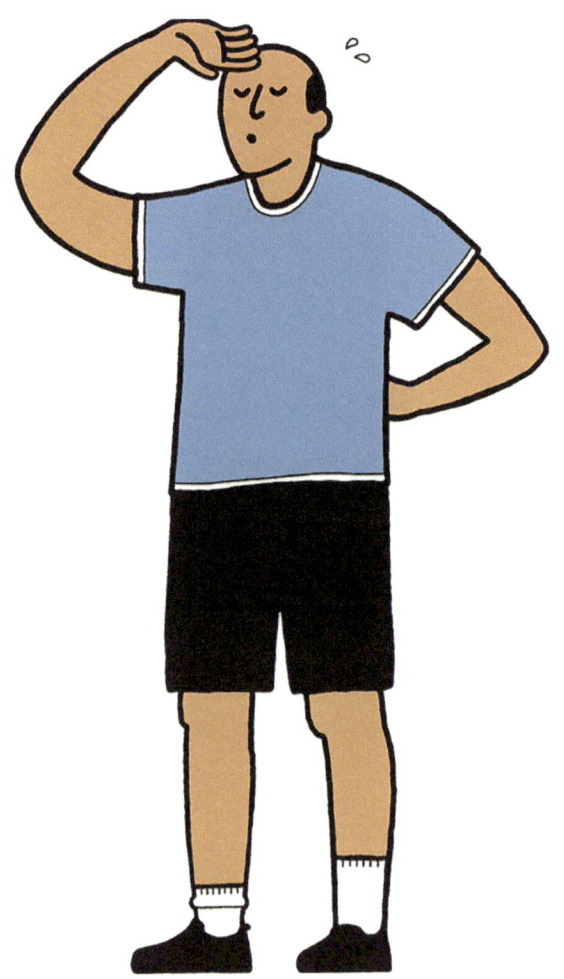

Value effort over natural talent

Putting in effort is far more important than natural talent because hard work is what leads to true success.[70]

So, seek challenge, focus on any small signs of the progress you are making, and take the time to celebrate small wins. 'Challenge' needs to be seen as an opportunity to learn and improve, not a way of proving yourself or testing how good you are already. Focus on improving, not proving.

"Hide not your talents, they for use were made. What's a sundial in the shade?"
Benjamin Franklin

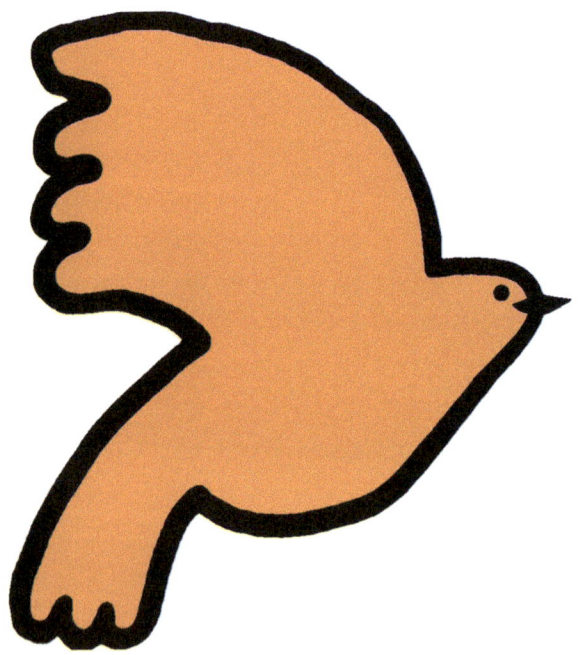

Adapt to the way others like to roll

Research shows that understanding diverse personalities leads to better communication and teamwork.[71]

To do this, first pay attention to how others prefer to interact: some for example may like direct communication while others prefer a gentler approach. Some might want to talk, others listen more. So 'dial up' their preference, and 'dial down' your own to adjust your style to match. This will make them feel it's far easier to trust and connect with you.

Watch out for those who have a very different preference to you – you are likely to find them annoying. Try not to think them stupid, or purposely irritating – they are probably thinking the same about you![72]

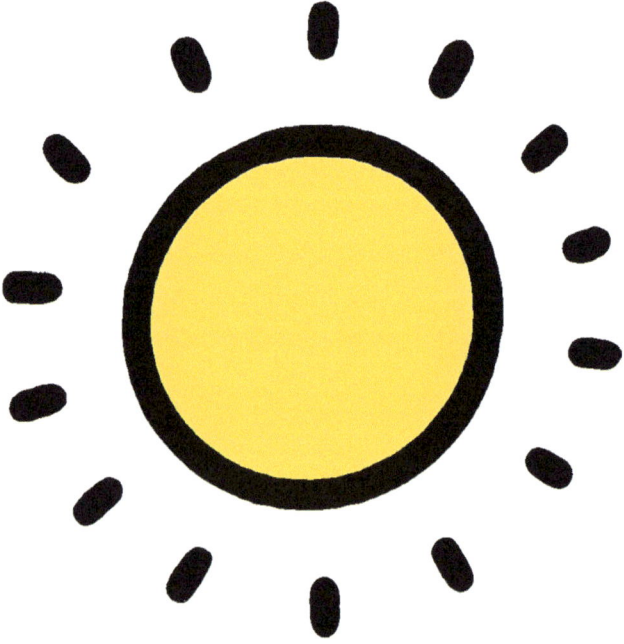

Engage in more joy-giving activities

This one action can reduce stress and anxiety, increase resilience, improve immune functioning, reduce pain, enhance creativity, improve brain health and even stave off dementia.[73] [74]

Write down all the things that make you feel great. Don't put the things you feel you should include. Think hard about what brings you joy deep down.

Read your list. As you do, think about what's most important in your life, and the things that are just not that important. What does this exercise tell you about how you are living your precious life right now? What should you be giving more time to… and less? We live an average of 4000 weeks… this fact can often help focus the mind on making sure we have more joy and less grind in our lives.

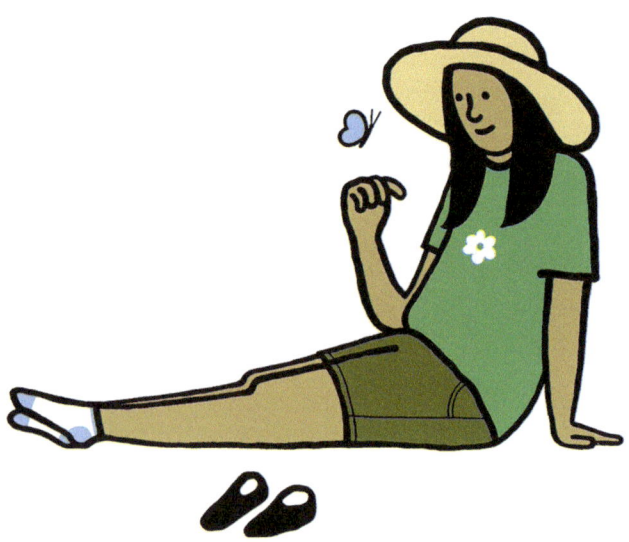

Spend time with Mother Nature

Whether she's in her green finery in the local park or forest, or the wondrous blue of a river, ocean or sky, nature will lower stress, improve mood and decrease rumination[75] – a key cause of poor mental health.[76] Even if you can't get out, watch a nature video as even this can be beneficial, leading to improvements in attention, positive emotions and the ability to reflect on a life problem.

Nature has inspired the practice of "forest bathing" or *shinrin-yoku* in Japan, where spending time in forests is a recognised form of therapy.

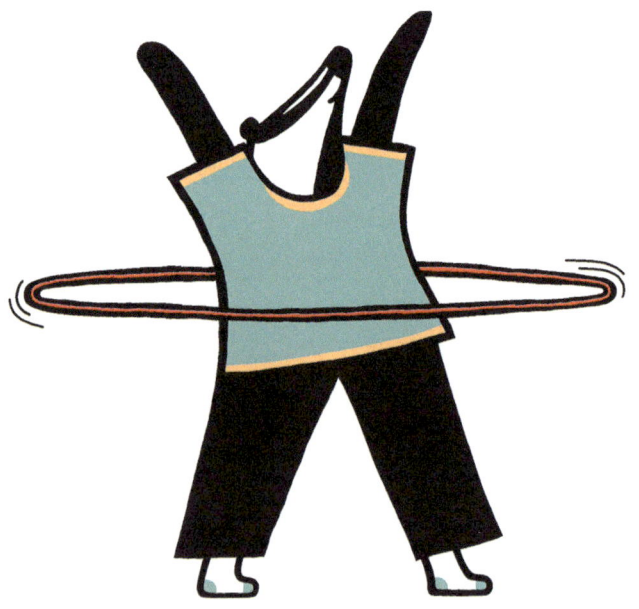

Move more

Regular physical activity will lower levels of anxiety and depression.[77] Sitting around all day will do the opposite and it's exhausting. Being sedentary goes against our evolutionary heritage.

As humans, we are designed to move a little bit almost all the time. Even small stretches and movements during the day can make all the difference.

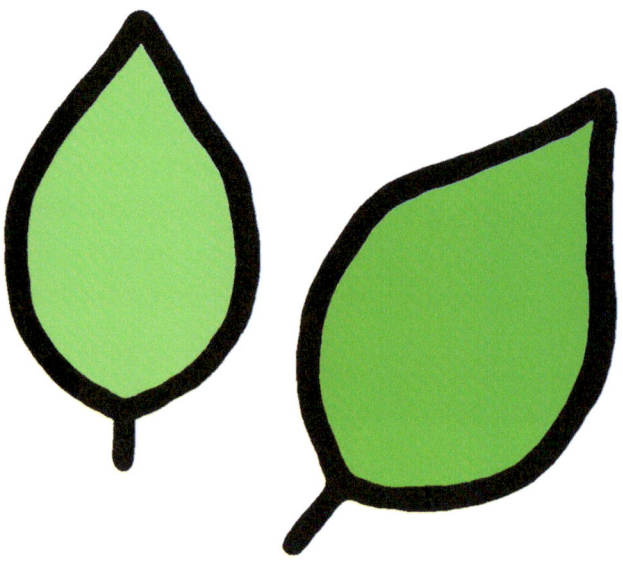

Treat stress as your friend

Stress is not always a bad thing. Eustress, a positive form of stress, releases adrenaline and cortisol, which heightens focus and energy, can make us sharper and more energised and so able to meet life's inevitable challenges.[78]

Next time you are feeling 'stressed', experiment by telling yourself that this is the biology of courage[79] and it's going to make you the best you can be.

"When you choose to view your stress response as helpful, you create the biology of courage."
Kelly McGonigal

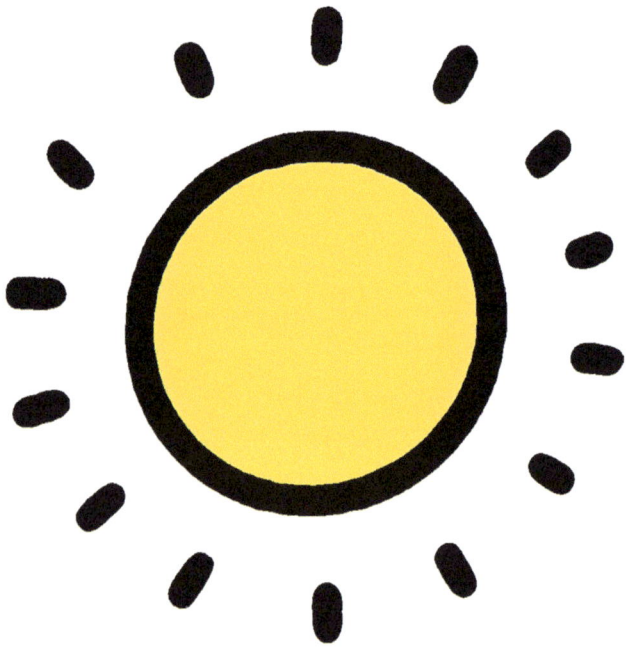

Ditch the show-face

Letting go of the "showface" and embracing vulnerability allows us to connect more honestly with ourselves and others. Research tells us that acknowledging and accepting emotional pain, rather than suppressing it is better for our health.[80]

Speaking from the heart, even when we need to be incredibly brave to do this, helps us understand our emotions and figure out where they have come from. Far better this, than sweeping emotions under the carpet or drowning them with alcohol or other forms of self-medication.

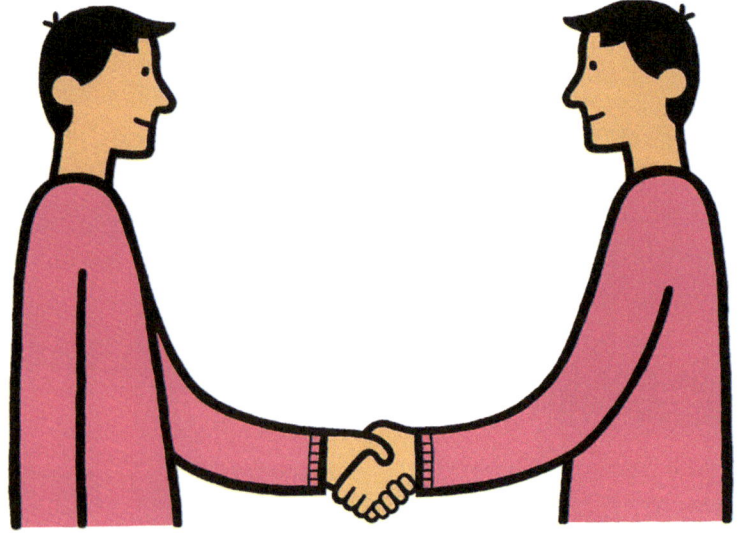

Accept

Accept, don't avoid your emotions and thoughts. By acknowledging and naming these without judgment, we allow ourselves to process them more fully and move towards healing.

This creates a deeper sense of connection with ourselves and a greater sense of well-being and clarity.[81] Research shows that acceptance reduces anxiety and increases resilience.[82]

This action might feel uncomfortable, but it could be the most important action we need to take to grow and discover ourselves during some of those darker days.

"The cave you fear to enter holds the treasure you seek."
Joseph Campbell

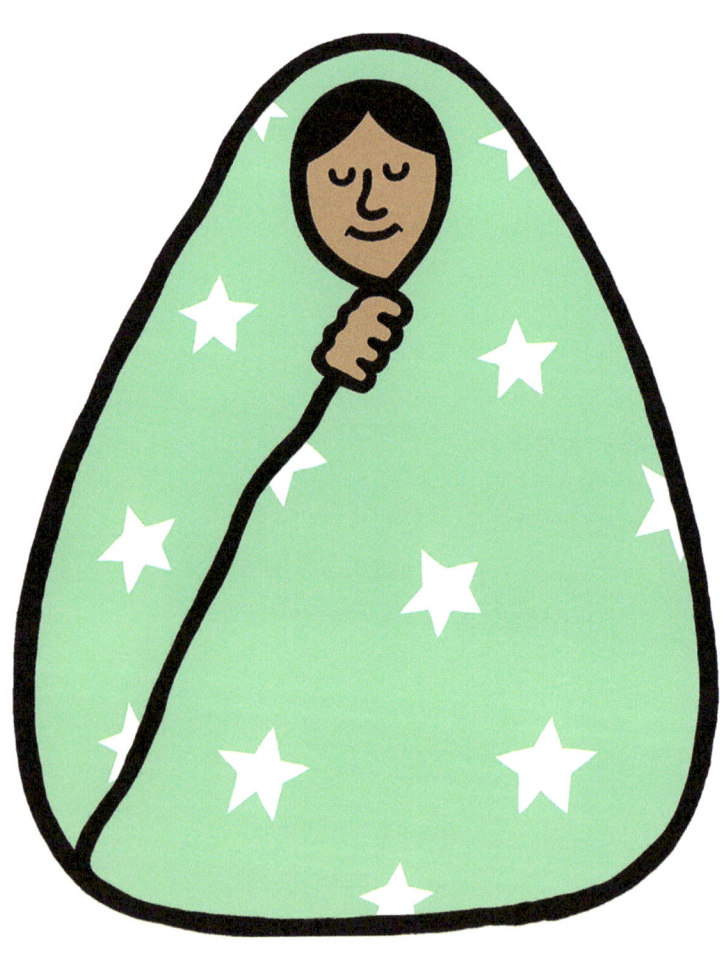

Prioritise feeling safe

All of us need to feel safe and secure. It is a core emotional need. If things around us are unpredictable or even dangerous then we will suffer.[83]

If you don't feel safe, ask yourself why. What is causing the feeling, and what could you and/or others do to fix this? If you can't change the cause, can you increase your strength in some way to make you feel safer?

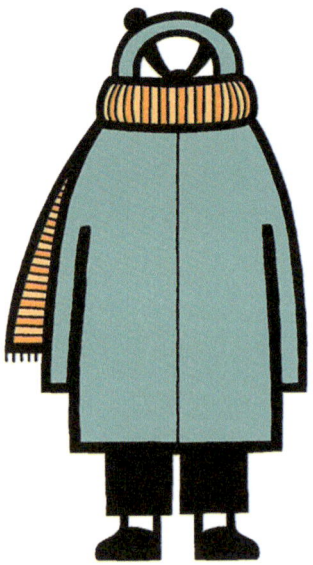

Stop dwelling on the bad stuff

Ruminating, or constantly replaying negative thoughts, traps us in a cycle of stress and worry. We ruminate in an attempt to solve problems or make sense of difficult emotions, but this serves to only deepen our distress.[84]

Practice noticing when you are going over and over things but getting nowhere, then write your thoughts down, read them back and focus on those things you can do something about – try and solve the problem, rather than dwell on the problem.

"As flies and such like vile creatures do never rest long upon smooth and fine polished places, but do stick fast to rough and filthy corners, so the murmuring mind does lightly pass over the consideration of all good fortune but never forgets the adverse or evil".

Justus Lupsius

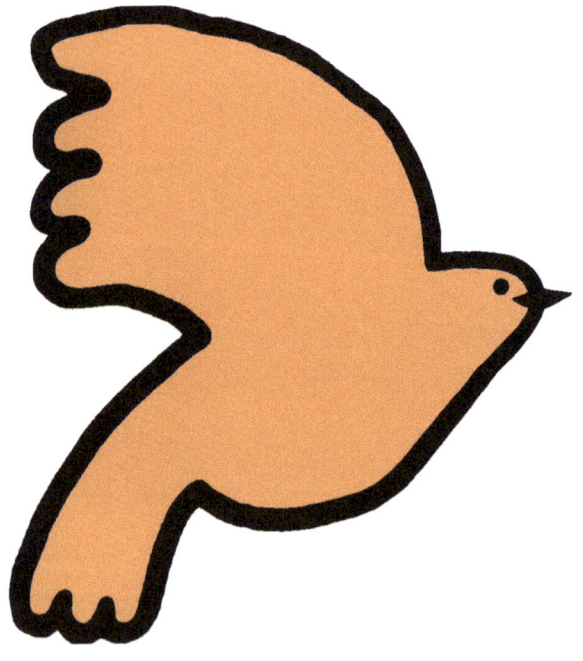

Stop people-pleasing

People-pleasing, putting others' needs over our own, is bad for our health.[85]

Many of us do it because we don't want to have to experience the horror of rejection or conflict, believing that constant approval will secure relationships. However, it often creates inner turmoil.

Setting healthy boundaries and practising assertiveness can reduce people-pleasing tendencies and improve emotional well-being. So, learn to say 'no' and start to regain control of your life.

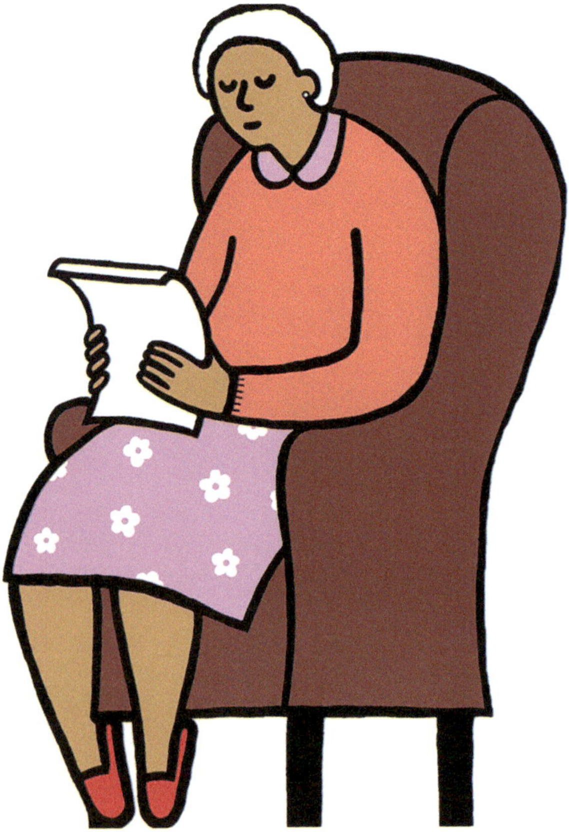

Pretend you are eighty

Writing a letter to yourself from the perspective of your 80-year-old self can be a great way of getting clarity on what truly matters.[86] This idea was inspired by Bronnie Ware, a former palliative care nurse who spent years listening to the regrets of her patients at the end of their lives[87].

In her work, Bronnie noted things she constantly heard from those nearing the end of their journey: wishing for the courage to live true to oneself, not working so hard, expressing feelings openly, maintaining close friendships, and allowing oneself to be happier.

Imagining yourself at 80, and writing a letter to the 'you' of today, often provides clarity on what truly matters in life.

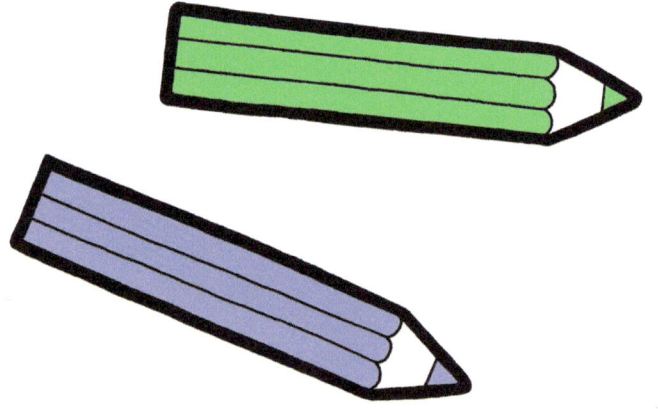

Let go of perfectionism

Research shows that perfectionism increases stress and lowers life satisfaction, usually because the standard is impossible to reach – we are always going to fall short of what we think we need to achieve to be happy.[88]

Being perfect often stems from the desire to avoid rejection, a habit created over years of being rewarded for getting things right, and perhaps punished for getting things wrong. Be more self-compassionate, strive for excellence, not perfection, and focus on the learning and effort you are making, not your shortfalls. Learn to know what good enough looks like, and if you don't know try asking others for their thoughts.

Around 1 in 5 adults struggle with perfectionism and this is linked to increased mental health challenges like anxiety and depression[89].

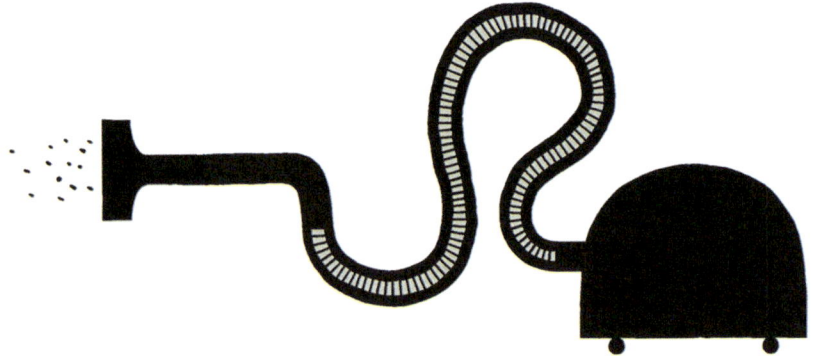

Avoid the mood hoovers

We catch moods as easily as we catch a cold. Where you can, spend time with people whose company you enjoy, who make you feel good about yourself – the radiators – and avoid those drains that suck the life out of you. Those we spend time with hugely influence our mood.[90]

Consciously surround yourself with supportive individuals and you create an environment that nurtures happiness. Simply cut the rope on those who don't. Remember – you have the choice. You'd never accept a bank account that you could only put money into and never withdraw from.

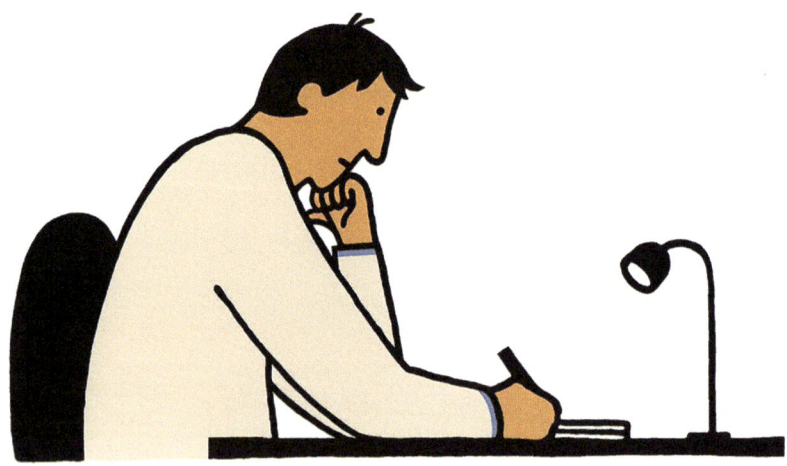

Book in some worry time

If you are a worrier, consider setting aside a specific time each day to note your worries in a diary. This is a good way of processing concerns and freeing up mental space for more positive thoughts.[91]

It also helps separate the stressors from daily life, reducing their impact. Recent research has found that doing this can lead to lower levels of anxiety and improved emotion regulation.

The average adult in the UK spends around 1 hour and 50 minutes per day worrying, with common worries including health, finances, and family.[92]

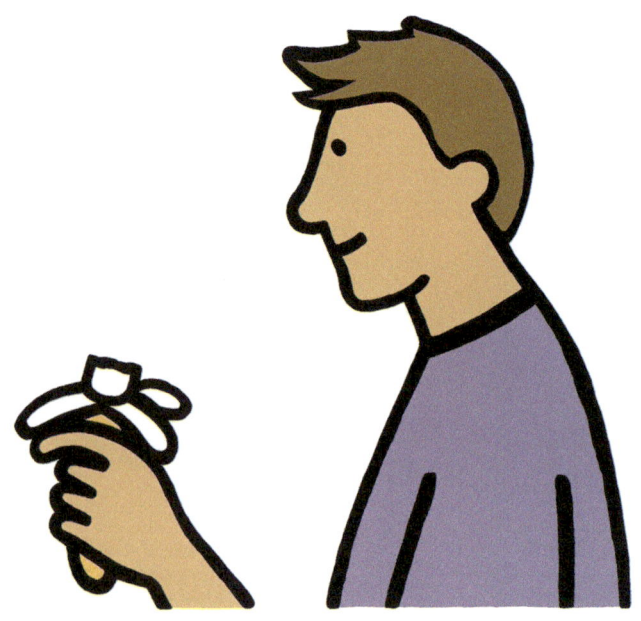

Have a banana!

Bananas contain tryptophan, a precursor to serotonin, and they are high in vitamin B6, which helps convert tryptophan to serotonin. The combination can provide a quick mood boost.[93]

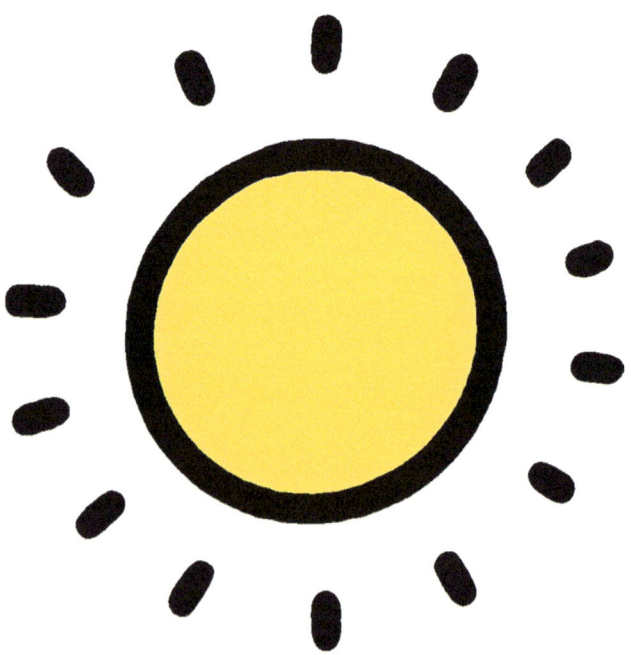

Act differently if feeling jittery

Anxiety is a misfire. Your brain telling you that your life is in danger. It isn't. It's a lie. You are not to blame. This is completely normal. You have a fine brain that is trying to look after you. To fix the misfire purposely find a situation that makes you feel a *little* anxious. Then behave as if everything is okay. This sends a message to the part of the brain that's triggering the 'get ready as I believe you might be in mortal danger' response that, well, you aren't.

When you sense your heartbeat thumping, the breathing becoming rapid and the stomach feeling like a washing machine, speak and move quietly and calmly, open out your posture, and even chew some gum. [94] This is a trick that tells the primate part of your brain that you are not in danger as you wouldn't be salivating, getting ready to eat, if you were in any real danger. Check out the other tips here, such as breathing deeply, laughing out loud and labelling your feelings to manage this misfire as just doing one of these will help you get back to a sense of safety and control.

Afterword

So, there we have it – practical, evidence-based tips to help you navigate life's ups and downs. Remember, it's the small, consistent actions that truly make a difference. Finding hope and calm in the storms is a lifelong journey, not a destination.

Choose the small actions that resonate with you and integrate them into your daily routine not just when you are experiencing a challenging time, but every day. This will make you stronger, more resilient and less likely to struggle when the inevitable storms of life hit. To stay on track, make these actions visible. Set reminders on your phone or screen saver, or use sticky notes on your fridge or mirror to show the principles you want to live by.

Try and make each action as enjoyable and easy as possible. Research suggests that habits tied to pleasure and ease are more likely to stick.

~~~

About Michelle Spirit

Michelle Spirit is a speaker, trainer, coach, visiting University lecturer and Licenced Insights Discovery® Practitioner, widely recognised as one of the UK's foremost experts on resilience and wellbeing.

Her career has encompassed mental health nursing, leadership development, coaching, and hypnotherapy. Over the past two decades, Michelle has partnered with organisations globally, working to create supportive environments where individuals and teams can find balance and so flourish.

Her collaborations include projects with **Mind**, the mental health charity, to enhance the resilience of Blue Light workers; **Microsoft**, where she facilitated workshops to deepen team understanding and connection; and **The University of Oxford**, helping to raise mental health awareness among staff and students. Additionally, she has supported countless professionals in high pressure, challenging roles, from social workers and GPs to teachers and nurses, equipping them with practical tools to help them thrive in the face of adversity.

Michelle lives in West Sussex, UK.

Acknowledgements

Special thanks to Niall Edworthy for your guidance and Mudd Bexley for bringing the ideas to life with such phenomenal creativity and care.

Finally, to the readers—this book is for you. Your journey motivates every word. Thank you for giving this book your time. I hope you find something in here that offers comfort, guidance and strength during life's more challenging moments.

Endnotes

1   Herzog, H. (2011). The Impact of Pets on Human Health and Psychological Well-Being. Current Directions in Psychological Science, [online] 20(4), pp.236–239. doi:https://doi.org/10.1177/0963721411415220.

2   Banks, M.R., Willoughby, L.M., and Banks, W.A. (2008). Animal-assisted therapy and loneliness in nursing homes: Use of robotic versus living dogs. Journal of the American Medical Directors Association, 8(3), pp.173-177. DOI: 10.1016/j.jamda.2007.11.007. Accessed 9 April 2020.

3   Wansink, B. and Sobal, J. (2007). Mindless Eating. Environment and Behavior, 39(1), pp.106–123. doi:https://doi.org/10.1177/0013916506295573.

4   Iyengar, S.S. and Lepper, M.R. (2000). When choice is demotivating: Can one desire too much of a good thing? Journal of Personality and Social Psychology, 79(6), pp.995–1006. doi:https://doi.org/10.1037/0022-3514.79.6.995.

5   Lepore, S.J. and Smyth, J.M. (2002). The writing cure: how expressive writing promotes health and emotional well-being. Washington, D.C.: American Psychological Association.

6   Harvard Health Publishing. (2020). The importance of having a sense of purpose. Harvard Medical School.

7   Harvard Health Publishing. (2021). How spirituality can enhance your health and well-being. Harvard Medical School.

8   Dunbar, R.I.M., Kaskatis, K., MacDonald, I. and Barra, V. (2012). Performance of Music Elevates Pain Threshold and Positive Affect: Implications for the Evolutionary Function of Music. Evolutionary Psychology, [online] 10(4), p.147470491201000. doi:https://doi.org/10.1177/147470491201000403.

9   P.Brickman, D.Coates and R.Jannoff-Bulman (1978). Lottery Winners and Accident Victims: Is happiness Relative? Journal of Personality and Social Psychology, 36, pages 917-27.

10   Rozin, P., & Royzman, E. B. (2001). Negativity bias, negativity dominance, and contagion. Personality and Social Psychology Review, 5(4), 296-320.

11   Steptoe, A., Deaton, A., and Stone, A.A. (2016). Subjective well-being, health, and ageing. The Lancet, 385(9968), pp.640-648. DOI: 10.1016/S0140-6736(13)61489-0.

12   Neff, K.D. (2011) 'Self-compassion, self-esteem, and well-being', Social and Personality Psychology Compass, 5(1), pp. 1–12.

13   Moser, J.S., Dougherty, A., Mattson, W.I., and Moran, T.P. (2017). Third-person self-talk facilitates emotion regulation without engaging cognitive control: Converging evidence from ERP and fMRI. Scientific Reports, 7(1). DOI: 10.1038/s41598-017-04047-3.

14   Neff, K.D. et al. (2020) 'Caring for others without losing yourself: An adaptation of the Mindful Self –Compassion Program for Healthcare Communities', Journal of Clinical Psychology, 76(9), pp. 1543–1562. doi:10.1002/jclp.23007.

15   Mullis, R. and Kera, G. (2023). Personal well-being in the UK, Office for National Statistics. Available at: https://www.ons.gov.uk/peoplepopulationandcommunity/wellbeing. Accessed 7 November 2023.

16   Hatori, K., et al. (2013) 'The effect of writing about the perceived benefits of interpersonal transgressions on psychological well-being in Japanese college students', Shinrigaku Kenkyu/Shinrigaku Kenkyuu, 84(2), pp. 156–161. Available at: https://doi.org/10.4992/jjpsy.84.156 (Accessed: 17 April 2024).

17   Louie, D., Brook, K. and Frates, E. (2016), The Laughter Prescription. American Journal of Lifestyle Medicine, [online] 10(4), pp.262–267. doi:https://doi.org/10.1177/1559827614550279.

18   Dunbar, R. I. M. (2014). Human Evolution: Our Brains and Behaviour. Cambridge University Press.

19   Csikszentmihalyi, M. (2013). Flow: The psychology of optimal experience. New York, NY: Random House.

20   Nehlig, A. (2013) 'The neuroprotective effects of cocoa flavanol and its influence on cognitive performance', British Journal of Clinical Pharmacology, 75(3), pp. 716–727. Available at: https://doi.org/10.1111/j.1365-2125.2012.04378.x.

21   Tan, C.-Y., Chuah, C.-Q., Lee, S.-T. and Tan, C.-S. (2021) 'Being creative makes you happier: The positive effect of creativity on subjective well-being', International Journal of Environmental Research and Public Health, 18(14), p. 7244. Available at: https://doi.org/10.3390/ijerph18147244.

22   Potthoff, J. and Schienle, A. (2021) 'Effects of self-esteem on self-viewing: An eye-tracking investigation on mirror gazing', Behavioral Sciences, 11(12), p. 164. Available at: https://doi.org/10.3390/bs11120164 (Accessed: 5 December 2021).

23   Chen, Y.-F., Huang, X.-Y., Chien, C.-H. and Cheng, J.-F. (2016) 'The effectiveness of diaphragmatic breathing relaxation training for reducing anxiety', Perspectives in Psychiatric Care, 53(4), pp. 329–336. Available at: https://doi.org/10.1111/ppc.12184.

24   Brown, R. P., & Gerbarg, P. L. (2013). Sudarshan Kriya Yogic breathing in the treatment of stress, anxiety, and depression: Part I—Neurophysiologic model. Journal of Alternative and Complementary Medicine, 19(1), 1-10.

25   Pennebaker, J.W. (1997) 'Writing about emotional experiences as a therapeutic process', Psychological Science, 8(3), pp. 162–166. Available at: https://doi.org/10.1111/j.1467-9280.1997.tb00403.x (Accessed: 5 March 2019).

26   Whillans, A.V., et al. (2017) 'Buying time promotes happiness', Proceedings of the National Academy of Sciences, 114(32), pp. 8523–8527. Available at: https://doi.org/10.1073/pnas.1706541114.

27   McAvoy, J. and Turley, M. (2016) Redemption. Pitch Publishing.

28   Weinhold, B.K. and Weinhold, J.B. (2014) How to break free of the drama triangle and victim consciousness. Colorado Springs, CO: Cicrcl Press.

29   Eger, E.E. (2020) The gift: Embrace the possible. New York: Scribner.

30   Pchelin, P. and Howell, R.T. (2014) 'The hidden cost of value-seeking: People do not accurately forecast the economic benefits of experiential purchases', The Journal of Positive Psychology, 9(4), pp. 322–334. Available at: https://doi.org/10.1080/17439760.2014.898316 (Accessed: 23 October 2020).

31 Gilovich, T., & Kumar, A. (2015). "We'll Always Have Paris: The Hedonic Payoff from Experiential and Material Purchases." Journal of Consumer Research, 42(1), pp. 29-44.

32 Dunn, E.W., Aknin, L.B. and Norton, M.I. (2008) 'Spending money on others promotes happiness', Science, 319(5870), pp. 1687–1688. Available at: https://doi.org/10.1126/science.1150952.

33 Hall, J.A., Taylor, S. and Smith, K. (2023) 'Quality conversation can increase daily well-being', Communication Research, p. 00936502221139363. Available at: https://doi.org/10.1177/00936502221139363.

34 Lieberman, M.D., Eisenberger, N.I., Crockett, M.J., Tom, S.M., Pfeifer, J.H. and Way, B.M. (2007) 'Putting feelings into words: Affect labelling disrupts amygdala activity in response to affective stimuli', Psychological Science, 18(5), pp. 421–428. Available at: https://doi.org/10.1111/j.1467-9280.2007.01916.x.

35 Fritzsche, B.A., Young, B.R. and Hickson, K.L. (2003) 'Individual differences in academic procrastination tendency and writing success', Personality and Individual Differences, 35(7), pp. 1549–1557. Available at: https://doi.org/10.1016/s0191-8869(02)00369-0.

36 Darki, C., Movahed, M. and Jaberi, A. (2022) 'The effect of classical music on heart rate, blood pressure, and mood', Cureus, 14(7). Available at: https://doi.org/10.7759/cureus.27348.

37 Huntington, C., Smith, P. and Adams, R. (2021) 'Happy, healthy, and wedded? How the transition to marriage affects mental and physical health', Journal of Family Psychology, 36(4). Available at: https://doi.org/10.1037/fam0000913.

38 Andrews-Hanna, J.R., Smallwood, J., and Spreng, R.N., (2014) 'The default network and self-generated thought: component processes, dynamic control, and clinical relevance'. Annals of the New York Academy of Sciences, 1316(1), pp.29-52.

39 Oettingen, G. (2015) Rethinking positive thinking: Inside the new science of motivation. New York, NY: Current.

40 Boggiss, A.L., Consedine, N.S., and Bishop, A.N. (2020) 'A systematic review of gratitude interventions: Effects on physical health and health behaviors', Journal of Psychosomatic Research, 135, p. 110165. Available at: https://doi.org/10.1016/j.jpsychores.2020.110165.

41 Emmons, R.A. and McCullough, M.E. (2003) 'Counting blessings versus burdens: An experimental investigation of gratitude and subjective well-being in daily life', Journal of Personality and Social Psychology, 84(2), pp. 377–389.

42 Harvard Medical School (2020) Importance of sleep: Six reasons not to scrimp on sleep. Available at: https://www.health.harvard.edu/staying-healthy/importance-of-sleep (Accessed: 15 October 2024).

43 RAND Corporation (2023) 'The societal and economic burden of insomnia in adults: An international study'. Available at: https://doi.org/10.7249/rra2166-1 (Accessed: 25 September 2023).

44 Bryant, F.B., Smart, C.M. and King, S.P. (2011) 'Understanding the processes that regulate positive emotional experience: Unsolved problems and future directions for theory and research on savoring', International Journal of Wellbeing, 1(1). Available at: https://doi.org/10.5502/ijw.v1i1.18.

45 Bryant, F.B., Smart, C.M. and King, S.P. (2005) 'Using the past to enhance the present: Boosting happiness through positive reminiscence', Journal of Happiness Studies, 6(3), pp. 227–260. Available at: https://doi.org/10.1007/s10902-005-3889-4.

46 Yang, C.-C., Gray, J.R. and Koenig, M.A. (2019) 'Alterations in brain structure and amplitude of low-frequency after 8 weeks of mindfulness meditation training in meditation-naïve subjects', Scientific Reports, 9(1), pp. 1–10. Available at: https://doi.org/10.1038/s41598-019-47470-4 (Accessed: 6 April 2020).

47 Kabat-Zinn, J. (2013) Full catastrophe living: Using the wisdom of your body and mind to face stress, pain, and illness. Revised edn. New York: Bantam Books.

48 Yang, C.-C., Gray, J.R. and Koenig, M.A. (2019) 'Alterations in brain structure and amplitude of low-frequency after 8 weeks of mindfulness meditation training in meditation-naïve subjects', Scientific Reports, 9(1), pp. 1–10. Available at: https://doi.org/10.1038/s41598-019-47470-4 (Accessed: 6 April 2020).

49 Zeidan, F., Johnson, S. K., Diamond, B. J., David, R. W., & Goolkasian, P. (2010). Mindfulness meditation improves cognition: Evidence of brief mental training. Consciousness and Cognition, 19(2), 597-605.

50 Snyder, C.R. and Lopez, S.J. (2001) Handbook of positive psychology. Oxford: Oxford University Press.

51 Kessler, R.C., Sonnega, A., Bromet, E., Hughes, M., & Nelson, C.B. (1995) 'Posttraumatic stress disorder in the National Comorbidity Survey', Archives of General Psychiatry, 52(12), pp. 1048-1060.

52 Statista (2023) 'Average daily screen time of adults in the United Kingdom (UK) in 2021 and 2022, by device'. Available at: https://www.statista.com/statistics/1191347/united-kingdom-average-daily-screen-time/.

53 Twenge, Jean M. "More Time on Technology, Less Happiness? Associations between Digital-Media Use and Psychological Well-Being." Current Directions in Psychological Science, vol. 28, no. 4, 22 May 2019, pp. 372–379, https://doi.org/10.1177/0963721419838244.

54 Vogel, E.A., Rose, J.P., Roberts, L.R. and Eckles, K. (2018) 'Social comparison, social media, and self-esteem', Personality and Social Psychology Bulletin, 44(5), pp. 673–688. Available at: https://doi.org/10.1177/014616721774419

55 Umberson, D. & Montez, J.K. (2010) Social relationships and health: A flashpoint for health policy. Journal of Health and Social Behavior, 51(Suppl), pp.S54-S66.

56 Gallup.com (2023) 'Almost a quarter of the world feels lonely', Gallup News. Available at: https://news.gallup.com/opinion/gallup/512618/almost-quarter-world-feels-lonely.aspx (Accessed: 24 October 2023).

57 Nagoski, E. and Nagoski, A. (2019) Burnout. New York: Ballantine Books.

58 Gallup (2021) State of the Global Workplace: 2021 Report. Available at: https://www.gallup.com

59 Bregman, R., Manton, E. and Moore, E. (2020). Humankind : a hopeful history. New York: Little, Brown and Company.

60 Dweck, C. (2016) Mindset: The New Psychology of Success. New York: Ballantine Books

61 Hammond, C. (2004) 'Impacts of lifelong learning upon emotional resilience, psychological and mental health: Fieldwork evidence', Oxford Review of Education, 30(4), pp. 551–568. Available at: https://doi.org/10.1080/030549804200030300 8.

62 Fields, R.D. (2008) The Other Brain. New York: Simon & Schuster.

63 Lawler, K.A., Younger, J.W., Piferi, R.L., et al. (2005). "A change of heart: Cardiovascular correlates of forgiveness in response to interpersonal conflict." Journal of Behavioral Medicine, 28(1), pp. 1-12.

64 Allemand, M., Job, V. and Christen, S. (2012) 'Forgivingness and subjective well-being in adulthood: The moderating role of future time perspective', Journal of Research in Personality, 46(1), pp. 32–39. Available at: https://doi.org/10.1016/j.jrp.2011.11.004 (Accessed: 25 October 2020).

65 Brown, B. (2013) Daring Greatly. London: Penguin UK.

66 Hall, L.H., Johnson, J., Watt, I., et al. (2016) 'Healthcare staff wellbeing, burnout, and patient safety: A systematic review', PLOS ONE, 11(7), pp. 1–12. Available at: https://doi.org/10.1371/journal.pone.0159015.

67 Dweck, C.S. (2006). Mindset: The New Psychology of Success. Random House.

68 Failory (2020) The Ultimate Startup Failure Rate Report. Available at: https://www.failory.com/startups/startup-failure-rate (Accessed: 30 October 2024).

69 Seligman, M.E.P. (2002). Authentic Happiness: Using the New Positive Psychology to Realize Your Potential for Lasting Fulfilment. Free Press.

70 Duckworth, A.L. (2016). Grit: The Power of Passion and Perseverance. Scribner.

71 Myers, I.B. (1995). Gifts Differing: Understanding Personality Type. Davies-Black Publishing.

72 Erikson, T. (2020) Surrounded by Idiots: The Four Types of Human Behavior and How to Effectively Communicate... With Each in Business - and in Life. St Martins Essentials.

73 Sheldon, K.M. and Lyubomirsky, S. (2006) 'Achieving sustainable gains in happiness: Change your actions, not your circumstances', Journal of Happiness Studies, 7(1), pp. 55–86. Available at: https://doi.org/10.1007/s10902-005-0868-8.

74 Williams, L.A., Schaefer, S.M., Rotman, B.L., Kober, H., Kross, E., Davidson, R.J. and Fredrickson, B.L. (2018) 'Reduced stress and greater well-being are associated with the frequency of positive emotions in daily life: Findings from the MIDUS national sample', Emotion, 18(6), pp. 901–910. Available at: https://doi.org/10.1037/emo0000320.

75 Mayer, F.S., Frantz, C.M., Bruehlman-Senecal, E. and Dolliver, K. (2009) 'Why is nature beneficial? The role of connectedness to nature', Environment and Behavior, 41(5), pp. 607–643. Available at: https://doi.org/10.1177/0013916508319745.

76 Bratman, G.N., Anderson, C.B. and Berman, M.G. (2012) 'The health benefits of nature experience: An emerging field of research', Frontiers in Psychology, 3, p. 340. Available at: https://doi.org/10.3389/fpsyg.2012.00340.

77 Rebar, A.L. and Stanton, R. (2019) 'Physical activity and mental health: A review of the literature', Psychology of Sport and Exercise, 16, pp. 204–214. Available at: https://doi.org/10.1016/j.psychsport.2014.04.001.

78 Cuddy, A. (2015). Presence: Bringing Your Boldest Self to Your Biggest Challenges. Little, Brown and Company.

79 McGonigal, K. (2015) The Upside of Stress: Why Stress is Good for You, and How to Get Good at It. New York: Avery.

80 Harvard Health Publishing. (2020). The healing power of vulnerability. Harvard Medical School.

81 Brach, T. (2019). Radical Compassion: Learning to Love Yourself and Your World with the Practice of RAIN. Viking.

82 Harvard Health Publishing. (2021). The power of emotional acceptance. Harvard Medical School.

83 Griffin, J., & Tyrrell, I. (2013). Human Givens: The new approach to emotional health and clear thinking. HG Publishing.

84 Querstret, D., Cropley, M., & Fife-Schaw, C. (2021). The effect of mindfulness-based stress reduction on rumination in individuals with anxiety disorders: A randomized controlled trial. Nature, 28(3), 654-662.

85 Brown, A. L., McKinley, C. J., & Wilson, C. (2021). The impact of boundary-setting on emotional health: A study of people-pleasing behaviors and their effects on well-being. Journal of Psychological Health, 46(2), 385-399.

86 Jones, A., Smith, T., & Williams, K. (2021). Reflective writing and its effects on rumination: A tool for mental clarity. Journal of Psychological Health, 48(3), 243-256.

87 Ware, B. (2012). The Top Five Regrets of the Dying: A Life Transformed by the Dearly Departing. Hay House.

88 Flett, G. L., & Hewitt, P. L. (2021). Perfectionism: A Relational Approach to Conceptualization and Measurement. Psychological Bulletin, 147(8), 781-794.

89 Mental Health Foundation (2021) Perfectionism and Mental Health. Available at: https://www.mentalhealth.org.uk (Accessed: 27 October 2024).

90 Holt-Lunstad, J., Smith, T. B., & Layton, J. B. (2022). Social Relationships and Mortality Risk: A Meta-analytic Review. PLOS Medicine, 19(2), e1003688

91 Schat, A. C. H., Van Woerkom, M., & De Lange, A. H. (2023). Worry Time: The Effects of a Structured Worry Intervention on Anxiety and Well-Being. Journal of Occupational Health Psychology, 28(1), 83-94.

92 Aviva (2018) The UK's biggest worries revealed. Available at: https://www.aviva.com/newsroom.

93 Parker, G., et al. (2013) 'Mood and carbohydrate intake: the serotonin hypothesis revisited', Nutrition & Neuroscience, 16(2), pp. 85–96. Available at: https://doi.org/10.1179/1476830512Y.0000000039.

94 Tyrell, M. (2024). 3 Instantly Calming CBT Techniques for Anxiety. Clear Thinking.

Printed and bound by CPI Group (UK) Ltd, Croydon, CR0 4YY

16/01/2025

01821190-0002